HOMOEOPATHY FOR EVERYDAY STRESS PROBLEMS

By the same author:-

Homoeopathic Medicine

The Homoeopathic Treatment of Emotional Illness

A Woman's Guide to Homoeopathy

Understanding Homoeopathy

Talking About Homoeopathy

An Encyclopedia of Homoeopathy

The Principles, Art and Practice of Homoeopathy

Emotional Health

Personal Growth and Creativity

The Side-Effects Book

HOMOEOPATHY FOR EVERYDAY STRESS PROBLEMS

A Guide to Better Emotional Health

by

Dr Trevor Smith
MA, MB, Bchir, DPM, MFHom

INSIGHT

Insight Editions
Worthing, Sussex
England

WARNING

The contents of this volume are for general interest only and individual persons should always consult their medical adviser about a particular problem or before stopping or changing an existing treatment.

Insight Editions
Worthing
Sussex
England

Published by Insight Editions 1993

© Trevor Smith 1993

Trevor Smith asserts the moral right to
be identified as the author of this work.

British Library Cataloguing in Publication Data

A catalogue record for this book is available
from the British Library.

ISBN 0-496670 19 6

Cover photograph by the author.

INTRODUCTION

In every family or work situation, some degree of stress occurs because of the demands posed by others and because people have different skills, abilities and levels of experience. The differences may create problems of rivalry, jealousy, resentment or envy. These can be positive as well as destructive, creating opportunities for new learning, new openings in terms of self-expression, challenge and potential growth. Stress only occurs when the fundamental differences between people are not accepted, or if competitive rivalry is excessive and inflexible, but especially where greater priority needs to be given to individual needs, interests and values.

Some tension forces are positive, an essential driving stimulus for motivation. They help to mobilise your excitement, the push and determination necessary for healthy success and goal-achievement.

Provided it is short term, focused and controlled, stress can be a constructive motivating force in your life. Adrenalin release, provides temporary energy for a highly-charged effort without faltering, stimulating increased muscular power, and cardiac output. When it is necessary to 'pull out the stops', some degree of stress pressure and frustration acts as a helpful stimulus to stamina and determination. But where the stress pressures are prolonged, they can quickly lead to 'burn-out', fatigue, insomnia, loss of concentration, and have a demoralising effect on your mind and body.

All forms of life are rhythmic, based on a two-tier model, with a positive high energy output phase (of contraction), followed by a negative one (of relaxation).

To maintain levels of energy flow, there must be a balance between positive muscular tone and the negative pause, or relaxation needs of the body. Both are essential for health. When they are in harmony, the individual is best able to cope with demands and challenges. But imbalance of either phase causes problems, either an excessive stimulation of mood (at a cost to output and productivity), or flattening, leading to anxiety, tension and loss of confidence.

The absence of stress or tonal force, creates a weak passive person, lacking drive, initiative and will-power. He may appear to be a cynical, long-suffering victim of events, or a jaded depressed personality who has given up trying or fighting for his beliefs. The effect is exactly similar to a state of depression associated with a post-viral M.E. syndrome, or following glandular fever.

Stress is a state of frustration and continual energy release going nowhere. This lack of direction may cause physical and emotional tension, frustration, exhaustion and anxiety.

When stress tensions become uncontrollable, sleep may also be affected. Problems remain because they have not been discussed or dealt with during the day. A combination of guilt, fear, frustration or anger, causes a restless shallow, interrupted sleep leading eventually to total exhaustion.

A stop-go mental existence tends to occur, with an urge to do something positive - tomorrow. There is usually a fundamental desire to make a new start:- a change in attitudes, to be more positive and outgoing, to be successful at something however small, in order to find a sense of self-respect. More often such praiseworthy intentions lead to nothing, because as soon as a problem arises, the inability to rest and relax undermines drive and endeavour.

'Living off your nerves' implies that the available energy for simple daily tasks is derived from adrenalin-release. The energy output is not easily controlled and quickly consumes all vitality. Energy loss occurs from excesses of the 'social' stimulants, especially coffee, tea and tobacco. After a quick and initial boost, it is almost impossible to sustain energy-output or 'staying power'. Because alcohol is a cerebral depressant, feelings of fatigue are considerably increased when alcohol is taken. There may be a high level of tension build-up, leading to depression.

Some occupations are more stressful than others. The type of work and the level of job satisfaction, or lack of it, plays an important contributory role in stress development. This is particularly a factor in emergency work where time is of essence. In this group 97% now suffer some form of stress symptoms, especially paramedics, such as ambulance workers. But stress plays a role in other occupations, including taxi-drivers with the pressures of uncertain employment, traffic and weather conditions, exposure to high levels of air pollution and little opportunity for exercise. Firemen and the police are constantly under pressure, never sure when they will have to face a crisis or horrific disaster.

Farmers are becoming increasingly stressed, no longer just affected by adverse weather conditions. Increasingly many are limited by financial pressures, and particularly small farmers are faced with major problems leading to stress and depression, (sometimes suicidal in intensity).

In complete contrast is the stress of the white collar executive. The harassed bank manager is faced with having to satisfy the financial needs of his clients and at the same time having to meet the stringent requirements of securities and guarantees demanded by his area manager. All of this can create enormous pressures and tensions which undermine health and relaxation.

If you have no job, have been made redundant, or uncertain employment, it is still important to keep this in perspective, allowing time and priority for the family and leisure; as well as discussion of the economic situation and finding training or work. If you are tired, under strain at work, it is not advisable to bring home work home from the office, or take on too much D.I.Y. projects. As far as possible, keep weekends free in order to look at and to share the needs of the family.

Regular breaks from home chores, a paced approach to pressure and demands, a rest period during the day, daily exercise of some kind, a wholesome diet low in fats and dairy products, avoiding alcohol, smoking, and excesses of tea or coffee, are all basic to family health, building up reserves to cope with stress and tension.

In any stress situation, distorted paranoid thinking may occur, especially when under heightened pressures. Try to recognize and minimize this type of thought activity because it undermines confidence and a balanced approach to problem solving. If your thinking is dramatic, persecuted, extreme, unreasonable, or dominated by fear, with high levels of anxiety and tension, it should be suspected as a possible factor undermining judgment. Usually paranoid thinking is short-lived and does not dominate the whole of thinking or take over the personality. It tends to become more balanced from explanation, discussion, humour, relaxation, and as the pressures are lifted.

A great deal of stress tension is caused by failure to communicate openly within the family. Too often there is inadequate or absent talking and failure to discuss the essential issues. This allows inappropriate fears to be perpetuated without balance or perspective.

It is important to listen to others, hear their opinions and life experiences, how they cope and approach a stress or pressure situation. Making the contact, sharing the fears, even to hear another persons point of view, helps clarify an area of anxiety and gives essential understanding to a situation which was previously vague. An argument or disagreement can also clarify a pressure situation, leading to a better feeling, clearer perspectives and aims for the future.

Stress may occur in any situation where relationships and people are involved, particularly at work, school, college, in the home, with neighbours, or the immediate family. When a pressure situation occurs, try to talk it through calmly, without suppressing any feelings that come up. Always directly express how you feel without giving way to either violence or flight, unless these are appropriate.

Most of us are not good at dealing with stress and some turn to violence, rejection, alcohol or withdrawal as a way out; particularly from extremes of feelings which are felt to be overwhelming. But silent unexpressed rage is also dangerous to health and often frightening. Learn to accept that you cannot win every situation and that an emotional crisis or pressure situation is often a way of motivating change in a stagnant situation. Self-control is an aspect of maturity, as long as it is does not deny emotion and feelings, with too much reasoned control.

If you are being abused or beaten if you try to talk and express your feelings, perhaps from a drunken or violent partner, a parent, step-parent or step-sibling, then you should not be talking in the immediate situation because it provokes violence. In such a situation, talking is too late, inappropriate or impossible, usually because it has been delayed too long.

Getting out of the relationship is the priority, perhaps to a 'safe' friend's house, community hostel, or social work care centre. You will still need to talk to a caring friend, member of the family or community, perhaps a social worker or member of the Samaritans about your feelings. Always discuss what has happened as soon as you feel safe and more secure.

7, Upper Harley Street
London NW1 4PS

Case reports

A man aged 35 worked for several weeks at a project, leaving home at 6.00 am and arriving at the office one hour before his staff. He worked late most evenings, working on the train going home and at weekends. He travelled widely, often arriving at the airport after a busy day to be met with a demanding problem. There were frequently evening meetings after his flight, continuing on until the early hours, and usually accompanied by a heavy meal and alcohol. His levels of stress were very high, mainly appearing as neck tension and rigidity. The neck muscles felt solid-like tree trunks. He drank beer regularly on the train home at night - just to keep going as he became increasingly exhausted. His weight increased from the beer intake and insufficient time for regular exercise. There was a slight but significant increase in blood-pressure and it was obvious that if he continued at this pace, he was a candidate for an early 'stroke' or heart attack.

A 60 year old man in the middle of a financial crisis, was under enormous pressure to complete the sale of his company before a deadline. At this time, he received an abusive telephone call from a former client, (who had lost money), threatening legal action. After the call, he became acutely excited and agitated, (taken over by paranoid thinking).He eventually rang the police, asking for protection, convinced the caller was lying in wait to attack or murder him. There was no reality in these fears and after discussing the threatening call with his family, he was able to perceive his own fears as a distortion and a stress reaction. He rapidly re-gained confidence and was highly amused at his over-reaction.

PSYCHOLOGICAL SYMPTOMS OF STRESS

Most people find these the most distressing feelings, and in some ways the most difficult areas to control and change. Irritability, tension and short-fuse reactions to pressure are very common stress symptoms. If allowed to gain hold over the individual, they may lead to fatigue and a loss or reduction of libido. Increased smoking and alcohol intake are other features.

If illegal drugs, such as marijuana or cocaine are used to gain either confidence or relaxation, intake may increase before they have any effect. 'Burn-out' is common. There is an increased risk of accidents too, especially when exercising or driving, due to impatience, faulty judgment of speed, and ignoring safety factors.

Relationship problems often reach a crisis, due to failure to listen, inability to comprehend another point of view, or lack of tolerance and understanding. There is an increased likelihood of divorce occurring at a time of intense stress pressures.

Any fatigue or weakness is aggravated by a troubled restless sleep with disturbing dreams or nightmares. Tension and tremor of the arms may cause hand-shaking in company. Panic attacks and extremes of emotion may also occur, similar to a young adolescent; with swings of mood from tears to laughter, rage or despair.

PHYSICAL SYMPTOMS OF STRESS

These symptoms are often the most obvious and embarrassing. They cause additional tension because it is felt that others will clearly notice the discomfort. Sweating, palpitations, headaches, indigestion with flatulence, acidity, nausea, peptic ulcer, pain and colicky spasm may occur, as the whole of the digestive process is undermined by excess acidity and a sluggish digestion. Many of the symptoms result from eating too much, too quickly, rather than chewing and tasting the food, and allowing time for healthy digestion to occur. Constipation or diarrhoea, sometimes a mixture of both, are common.

Backache (low back syndrome) is a painful complication, due to tension and spasm of the long muscles of the spine because of stress intensity, failure to relax, and quick ill-timed reactions and movements. A frozen shoulder, or limitation of movement with pain due to spasm, may occur in the upper back, neck and shoulder blade area.

Eczema is a common, often variable, chronic symptom, the skin dry, itchy, and infected from the intense scratching that is invariably present. Asthma, colitis (frequently diagnosed as Irritable bowel syndrome), a chronic explosive watery or loose diarrhoea, with blood and mucus on the stool, is common. Hoarseness with laryngitis, leading to complete or partial loss of voice may be of stress origin, or the pitch of the voice may become weak and unreliable in any public or pressure situation due to fear and loss of confidence. A vocal chord may be paralysed for months until the stress situation is finally resolved.

Raised blood-pressure (hypertension) is often stress-related, associated with a high fat or protein diet, excessive salt and carbohydrate intake with increased weight. Emotional tension is frequently the underlying reason for compulsive dieting, alternating with binge eating, especially craving chocolate bars or cakes, wine or beer. The artificially high sugar intake may lead to eczema, acne, or chronic fungal skin problems. Anal itching (or pruritis ani) is another common problem associated with a high sugar intake, excessive sweating, poor personal hygiene and suppressed irritation. The scratching is sometimes the only apparent sign of the inner turmoil and feelings of pent-up rage and anger. Prostatic or bladder problems may also be stress-related.

Post-viral M.E. syndromes with collapse and weakness are common stress manifestations, with almost total exhaustion, lack of concentration or drive, and variable muscle pains which defy diagnosis or fail to consistently improve with any form of conventional treatment.

Tight chest discomfort is a common stress symptom, causing shortness of breath, exacerbating asthma and wheezing in tense or pressure situations.

Stress is an important factor in irregular or painful period problems, recurrent infections (including thrush, colds, sore throat, and sinusitis), various allergies, for example hay-fever and asthma. It is usually the major underlying cause of many distressing sexual problems for men and women.

HOMOEOPATHY AND STRESS

Homoeopathy acts deeply and profoundly upon the mind, helping to loosen rigid defensive patterns of thinking, and releasing blocked areas of repression. These include emotions and memories, together with their intrinsic (bound-up) energy, which in the past have undermined physical health and drained energy reserves.

Because homoeopathy acts to restore order and balance, it also loosens emotional knots and 'no-go' areas within the mind, helping to recall and free past traumas and hurts to conscious memory. They can then be thought about in a different, more mature way. The homoeopathic potency will also liberate a more spontaneous expression of feelings, allowing a healthier relationship to flourish and grow. It supports the ability to more openly acknowledge love, caring, and need, as well as hurts which were often denied in the past.

Homoeopathy promotes relaxation by reducing tension and treating it's fundamental cause. It promotes a balanced rhythmic approach to life, rebuilding vital energy reserves, and encouraging a relaxed frame of mind. It also helps to restore the sleep rhythm as the mind becomes less active at night.

By reducing tension and irritability, problems can be more easily discussed and resolved. This leads to the possibility of new insights developing, a lessening of self-destructive guilt, more balanced judgements and greater confidence.

ADVICE ON TAKING HOMOEOPATHIC REMEDIES

Sources of remedies

The remedies recommended throughout the book should be purchased directly from a homoeopathic pharmacy or health shop. Always ensure that your remedies are from a reliable source and take them in the sixth centesimal or 6c potency.

Using the remedies

The potencies or strengths, come as small round pills or tablets, made of sucrose (or lactose). If you are sensitive to lactose, you should order your remedies directly from a homoeopathic pharmacy, requesting a sucrose or lactose-free pill base for the remedies. Because the medicine, or homoeopathic dilution is applied directly to the surface of the pill, they should not be handled. They are best placed directly into the mouth from the lid of the container, and sucked under the tongue. They should always be taken at least 20 minutes before or after food or drink (except water); orthodox medicines; vitamin or mineral supplements; and toothpaste.

Substances to avoid

Do not drink peppermint tea when taking homoeopathic remedies. Avoid coffee, tea, and cocoa, because their high caffeine content may diminish their effect.

Keeping the remedies fresh and active

The medicines should be stored in a cool, dry, dark area, away from strong odours, especially camphor, oil of wintergreen, perfume, essential oils, after-shave, and soap. In this way, their action will last indefinitely.

Diet and alcohol

A bland diet is recommended, not eating to excess, or using strong spices. Alcohol should be avoided, and smoking reduced or stopped altogether during treatment, especially for lung, heart, or circulatory problems.

How long should remedies be taken for

Remedies should be taken for as long as any symptoms persist - and then stopped. If new symptoms arise during homoeopathic treatment, they should be watched carefully, especially if they have occurred in the past. The homoeopathic action may sometimes cause earlier symptoms to reappear. They are usually fleeting, but if persistent, they will require a new remedy.

Aggravation of symptoms

An aggravation of symptoms, after taking the remedies, is a positive sign and means the potencies are working well. It is usually short-lived, and does not undermine the overall sense of well-being and improved vitality.

Side-effects

If you use them correctly, there are no side-effects or risks from homoeopathy. If you take a wrong remedy, or a whole box of the pills, they will cause no harm. The remedies can be safely used during pregnancy, breast-feeding, or given to the youngest baby.

Homoeopathy and orthodox medicines

The remedies do not interact with orthodox medicines, or undermine their action. If you are given a course of antibiotics, it is best to stop homoeopathic remedies for this period. Some orthodox drugs, especially steroids, may reduce or neutralise the homoeopathic effect.

17

Pain

Homoeopathy will help with some types of pain and spasm, but it is not the treatment of choice for very acute or severe pain, and if this occurs, orthodox treatment is recommended.

Homoeopathy and the age of the patient

Homoeopathy acts at every age, the reaction varying with age, strength, and the intrinsic resistance or vital energy reserves of the patient. It acts very quickly in a child, or fit young person, but is much slower in an elderly person, particularly if old, weak, or feeble.

Homoeopathy and acute illness of the elderly

It is often better initially, to give an orthodox treatment to an elderly person during an acute illness. If possible, use homoeopathy when convalescent, and before severe weakness occurs.

Safety of the homoeopathic approach

Homoeopathy is nevertheless helpful in the older age group:- for muddled thinking, poor memory, insomnia, restlessness, anxiety or tension problems. It does not cause confusion of the mind or agitation, which may be a severe problem when some orthodox drugs are used.

ACCIDENT PRONENESS

This is a common problem for all stress sufferers, especially when high levels of anxiety and tension have been allowed to build-up and accumulate to the extent that they undermine:- co-ordination, balance, fluency and ease of movement, the ability to judge speed and position, also spacial perspective as far as it concerns risk or danger.

When the nerves are frayed, to the extent that any movement carried out is a tense one, there is little chance of relaxation during the day and every exercise or body movement is a tense one with too much adrenalin and heightened tone, making the muscles prone to damage. It is particularly likely to occur whenever a competitive sport is carried out, with a very high risk of tendon injury (usually a tear or painful spasm), sometimes a dislocation, especially tennis elbow, frozen shoulder, or an acute low-back problem.

But accident proneness is likely to occur in any situation, not just those on the tennis court or in the gym. Almost any activity can lead to an injury or accident. Simply bending down, may cause the back to suddenly 'lock', requiring several weeks or months of bed-rest because of paralysing agony due to spasm of the powerful dorsal muscles along the spine.

Other symptoms happen when eating. Choking may occur, or a bowel or digestive upset. The problem may manifest as just being clumsy, spilling the drinks, dropping a supper dish, breaking plates, or throwing away the silver knives together with the fruit peelings into the bin, losing keys, important documents, forgetting an overdue bill, or to give instructions to a child or colleague, and putting letters into the wrong envelopes. There are especial high-risk dangers in the garden, when using power tools, a hammer or saw, involved in D.I.Y. home improvements, using a ladder, walking the dog or from equestrian pursuits.

Car accidents are particularly common when stressed, especially if feeling frustrated, resentful or angry. Driving a new car close to home, when the usual care and attention is forgotten and stress preoccupations take over, is a particularly vulnerable time. Detailed concentration is often undermined for several months following a divorce or separation. The inevitably hurt, highly intense feelings, together with aggression and often deep caring, may lead to stiffness and anger at the wheel, unreliable on the brake or accelerator pedals.

Character traits which aggravate the condition
Impatience, rushing to the extent of being off-balance both physically and emotionally. Too intense, trying to do too much, over-zealous and excessively competitive, caring too much about approval and pride.

Practical steps to improve things
Slow down. Don't fill every minute with activity. Take more time to sense and feel what is the right position for you to feel comfortable and at ease. Try to sense the natural space between you and others. Once found, take care not to cramp or exclude it. Realise that you don't have to win at everything or to be perfect to gain love and approval. Enjoyment and participation counts just as much as winning. Be natural and do what you can at any moment of the day, staying in touch with what **you** want and who **you** are.

Remedies to consider:-

Aconitum
For acute stress problems caused by fear or a sudden shock.

Agaricus
Clumsiness is associated with fear, often covered up by constant talking and yawning.

Bovista
Mainly a female remedy, with tearful irritability, poor levels of concentration, constantly dropping things, and making mistakes when writing.

Calcarea
There is poor spatial awareness and co-ordination, coupled with sluggish weakness. Sweating, especially of the head is common.

Causticum
There is peevish irritability with depressive mood swings and lack of confidence. Anxious uneasy moods. The hands may develop a tremor, or become weak, with a tendency to drop things.

Colchicum
The mood varies from anxiety to irritability, the hands weak, with a marked tremor.

Ipecacuanha
The mood is one of impatience and short-fuse irritability. Nausea and weakness are marked.

21

Kali carb

Lack of energy and sluggishness aggravates any anxiety problems. Most of the problems are worse in the early morning hours.

Lachesis

All the symptoms are worse after sleep, with intolerance of tight clothing and 'verbal diarrhoea'.

Lycopodium

The personality appears much more mature and independent than in reality. The accidents are usually due to a tendency to anticipate everything and to want to rush at every situation.

Nux vomica

Spasms of short-fuse irritability, everything in life over-intense, rushed or excessive. Injuries tend to occur in sports as he hates losing and is very competitive.

Pulsatilla

Movements, like the emotions are dramatic to the point of being extreme and hysterical. It is the wide variability and extremes of reaction which causes accidents.

Sulphur

The individual is not at his best in the mornings, unable to negotiate the most obvious objects. Heat aggravates the clumsiness, which is apparent in everything he does. Life is never smooth, full of snags and constant pitfalls.

AGITATION

Agitation is excessive fear or anxiety translated into restless movement and pacing. Like a tiger in a cage, one moment you may be lying down, the next one up and having to keep moving in order to maintain control. The whole body is too taut like a tightly wound up spring, at times bent over with spasm, jack-knifing the body into odd contours to find rest and relaxation. If the pacing is more internal, the restlessness within the mind, the feeling and thought processes are never still, not even in sleep, because the dreams contain themes of terror, persecution, pressure or fear. Thoughts jump from one area of anxiety to another, but always to extremes, fearing or anticipating disaster.

Stress agitation is usually controllable and of short duration, often relieved by contact with others and by reassurance. It does not constitute an illness in itself. The agitation is usually part of an overall situation of anxiety and often loss of confidence, fear of not coping, having to meet others, a change of routine, or any situation when on display, being judged, or in public.

Case reports
A husband took early retirement and insisted on going everywhere with his wife, including shopping. She became agitated, knowing that because of his deprived background, he always buys far more than they need - several pounds of fruit when she would have bought single items or just enough for the next few days. This made her feel agitated, as she knew he would not listen and quickly becomes irritable. Also she hates an argument. As a result she become overwhelmed with mixed feelings - resentment, frustration, impatience,

guilt and anger; enraged that she would have to cope with the extras, to cook more. She felt under pressure and agitated, yet unable to express her mounting rage.

A financial executive, in charge of a busy office became pressurised and agitated because of a meeting with a client who was bringing a new important account. A morning meeting was planned with lunch at a nearby restaurant. He became increasingly agitated and nervous, mainly fearing being unable to cope socially with the lunch; eating with them, wondering if he could stay the course until the afternoon without the agitation showing by sweating; feeling weak, or having to rush out for fresh air; perhaps leave the meeting or even the office to rush home to find relief from pressure and some security. All of this created tension, adding pressure to the business of the day.

Character traits which aggravate the condition
There are poor controls over emotions, far too sensitive, over-reacting, getting quickly excited, expecting perfection; really too much of everything, and then getting disappointed or hurt. There are problems of staying in touch with the real self, needs, aims, and directions, also staying emotionally centred.

Practical steps to improve things
Keep all your emotions more in balance, not allowing yourself to react excessively to either success or disappointment. Practise staying on an even keel, calm and relaxed whatever the provocation or outcome. Stay in touch with your essential self, personal gifts and achievements. Avoid creating disasters and dramas out of life's vicissitudes. Try to meditate at times of great disappointment or frustration, and relax more.

Remedies to consider:-

Arsenicum   Anguish, restlessness, and excitability with fear are marked, usually worse after midnight.

Belladonna   The face is red, excitability marked. A tendency to rage and bite when in a mood of violent fury.

Hyoscyamus   A remedy for violent states of agitation with intolerance and mistrust.

Lycopodium   The agitation is always concerned with what might happen, fear of the future, especially worse in the afternoon and early evening.

Natrum mur   Anxiety with agitation, weakness, a depressive mood, often tearful.

Phosphorus   The agitation is due to fear and apprehension, with a constant need for reassurance and comfort.

Silicea   A useful remedy for stress agitation when due to lack of confidence.

Zinc met   There is talkative, excitable restless behaviour, mainly in the evening.

AGORAPHOBIA

Fear of open spaces is a common stress problem with loss of confidence and security outside a narrow 'safe' area, usually near to home or work. Anxiety occurs in situations involving driving, especially in the country, where there are panoramic views, or the road seems to run on forever like an endless ribbon, threatening to engulf or swallow one up, taking you further away from safety and security. Distances seem vast and immeasurable. It may seem impossible to get home again, or there is fear of collapsing at the wheel, having an accident, a malaise, or just a panic feeling with no one to help and far from home. It is not surprising that it is possible to dread losing control, or in some way overwhelmed with frightening, unspeakable feelings.

Such paralysing and incapacitating thoughts are not just confined to the motor car and may involve any form of transport, including travel by air, train, underground and sometimes going down an escalator. Often the fears are worse in crowds, especially where there is any delay or hold-up, for example at the supermarket check-out, a queue, or hold-up on the motorway. Exasperation is combined with a sense of being trapped and unable to get out of a situation, for example, off the road when on a motorway. Such hold-ups lead to fear of loss of control and violence, with a desperate need to run away, but nearly always linked to a sense of losing contact with what is familiar, or imminent collapse.

Much of the problem relates to anxiety about being free, more independent, and assertive. There are usually strong ties to the family, often with childish anxieties, an over-dependent marriage and similar relationships

26

with others. The fears experienced are often a powerful compromise between strong wishes to be more outgoing, creative, assertive, different, with needs to continue old patterns and ties, although these limit the personality, personal achievement, happiness, and stifle development and growth.

Case report
A woman in her 50's lost her husband from a sudden heart attack. The marriage had always been happy, but she tended to be over-dependent on him. A year before he died, the couple were involved in a near-miss accident on the motorway and had swerved to avoid a lorry. Since his death, the dread of having a fatal accident replaced her grief at losing her partner and she became dominated by this earlier fear, making her terrified of driving anywhere other than in the immediate proximity of the house.

Character traits which aggravate the condition
A tendency to keep feelings suppressed, locked tightly down, with fear of being open and exposing emotional needs. Fear of anger and violence, irritated and losing control in situations requiring a cool head and patience.

Practical steps to improve things
See the basic problem as fear of facing up to inner needs, drives and feelings, and try honestly to confront these, to get to know them better. Once you are more in touch with yourself, slowly increase your exposure to the phobic or fear areas, adding to this as you become more clear about those aspects you are suppressing. Challenge the reality and assumptions (the risks and dangers), of the agoraphobic situation, as you become more open and confident with yourself.

Remedies to consider:-

Aconitum Acute fear is the main cause of the phobic problem. Agitation is usually a marked feature.

Argentum nit This is a very useful remedy for agoraphobic problems, especially when there is fear of a future situation involving other people, and being the centre of attention. All symptoms are worse for heat.

Gelsemium Fatigue, sluggish apathy and exaggerated often dramatic fears. Useful for mild phobic problems.

Natrum mur Depression is a feature with tearful anxiety and exhaustion. Always feels worse for social contacts.

Phosphorus There is a high level of anxiety, with restless excitable moods and impatience.

Pulsatilla All symptoms are variable, worse for heat or cold. The moods are dramatic, variable, and usually tearful.

Silicea For chilly states of weakness and exhaustion, lacking in confidence and drive.

ALCOHOL AND STRESS

Alcohol in controlled moderation is enjoyable and a relaxing pastime, which most people indulge in from time to time. It only becomes a problem when alcohol is seen as the only way to obtain relief from anxiety, lack of confidence, or depression.

It is often used to try to resolve a shyness or depressive problem, particularly one where communication and conversation is a problem. But because alcohol is a cerebral depressant it tends to worsen confidence problems rather than helping to solve them. It weakens drives to be more self-expressive, the determination to go out and meet people. After an initial and often temporary relaxation of tension, a loss of inhibition occurs within the immediate social situation but which does not lead to any lasting psychological confidence and growth. This is because apparent confidence is acquired at the expense of alcohol dependency, rather than based on experience and overcoming fear or inhibitions. A compulsive alcohol intake, quickly becomes an entrenched habit, undermining physical energy and health, often with weight gain from the extra fluid and sugar intake. This combined with loss of appetite from gastritis, liver irritation and eventually damage, may lead to permanent indigestion problems. Psychologically, alcohol leads to a jaded sense of precarious well-being, quickly leading on to fatigue, withdrawal, remoteness, irritability of mood and depression.

The ability to communicate and to share is not helped by the alcohol habit. It is usually a self-indulgent, comforting process, based on flight, which isolates you

29

from the major problem area, the personalities involved, the areas of conflict, and leads to lack of confidence. Because of its depressant central nervous action, alcohol also undermines any real and useful personal interaction, the quality of self-expression, sharing, and communication.

Because alcohol causes addiction and dependency, it weakens the personality, controls, eventually insight, and the ability to perceive why problems occur, and the real causes of difficulties and how best to remedy and resolve them.

Character traits which aggravate the condition
There is a tendency not to deal with anxiety and frustration as it occurs, denying feelings, or allowing them to fester and expand beneath the surface. As a result, intrinsic energy tends to re-emerge more violently. Alcohol is often used as a substitute for more open spontaneous expressions, a way of suppressing feelings and reactions, at the same time also suppressing individuality in a self-destructive way.

Practical steps to improve things
Practise more open, frank self expression with much greater spontaneity. Spend more time talking about needs, hurts and feelings, remaining calm and not becoming abusive. Slowly restrain the use of alcohol. In situations of frustration, practise discussing your feelings and reactions as soon as you are aware of them. Try to develop an alternative outlet for rage and frustration, for example:- going for a long walk, working in the garden, relaxation, meditating, just straight talking to the people you care about, and who are involved in your life and emotions.

30

Remedies to consider:-

Agaricus Useful for acute alcoholic states, with confused, excitable, talkative behaviour, as occurs in D.T.'s. Giddiness and headache from alcohol excess.

Avena sat There is a combination of exhaustion, restless insomnia, and inability to concentrate, the memory poor. A useful remedy for long standing alcoholism.

Nux vomica There is anger and short-fuse irritability, also long standing digestive problems with heartburn and nausea.

Sepia The alcohol problem is mainly the result of evening exhaustion, dragged down by pelvic or abdominal discomfort. Feels indifferent to others and is extremely irritable.

Sulphur A useful remedy for long-standing problems, with early morning diarrhoea, chronic indigestion problems, confusion of thinking, and skin rashes or areas of infection.

ANOREXIA

Eating may have been a preoccupation over the years, the emphasis on dieting followed by periods of binge eating and self-indulgence. There is often an unhealthy preoccupation with being slim, on losing weight, how to prevent a protruding paunch or stomach, or middle-age spread. The emphasis is always on appearance, eternal youth, fitness and beauty, to the exclusion of more meaningful creative experiences in life. Stress anorexia does not however take over the whole person as in anxorexia nervosa, or lead to severe illness, a very low body weight, and bulimia or compulsive self-induced vomiting. Life may become dominated by a hypochondriacal preoccupation - how to control the appetite, being constipated, what to eat and what not to. In many ways the preoccupation with detail and appearance is a flight from closer contact with others, often hiding deeper feelings of loss, depression, loneliness, and unhappiness. Many of the feelings of loss and loneliness date from early childhood, often since separation from a partner, close friend, or sibling, who was deeply cared for and brought warmth, comfort and happiness. For others, the loss was of a much loved pet, sometimes a parent or grandparent. Mood swings and tearfulness are common, with dependency on a prescribed stimulant or tranquilliser.

Psychologically there is a sense of being bloated, fat unattractive or ugly. The self image is described as podgy, squat, and dumpy, sometimes all front, tummy or thighs, and often not tall enough. Such critical and punishing self-imagery, often dates from teasing since childhood by other children and has 'stuck', leading to confidence loss, feelings of inadequacy and depression.

Character traits which aggravate the condition

There is a tendency to be rigid, to put far too much emphasis on the opinion of others and their judgments. Too much time is given to appearance, body size, and food, rather than the quality and style of life, what **you** want to do, and excuses why it is not possible, rather than why it is. The control of food intake and body weight is given an undue prominence, keeping the body slim, narrow and thin. In the same way feelings and reactions, needs and emotions are kept within a tight narrow anorexic band which you control. But all of this creates problems, denies the essential you, creates a trapped resentful feeling, not allowing the true self to emerge and grow. It is the essence of you which fundamentally is kept at near starvation point.

Practical steps to improve things

Try to allow yourself much more variation of social contacts and of food. Stop weighing yourself, and throw the scales away. Eat sensibly, but always eat good quality wholesome food, eating when you are hungry. It is better to eat three small meals a day until your appetite returns, or you will become ravenous after 2-3 hours and be tempted to binge on junk food, start to feel guilty, and then get back into dieting again. Try to break the old rigid patterns and let yourself be a much more free, emerging individual. Sense the excitement of movement and growth, but don't restrict it; seeing that you matter, that your life matters, and that it is a precious thing which should not be restricted or abused. If you feel angry and resentful inside, try to trace back the origins of the feelings and look at them with adult eyes, not trying to change the emotions.

Remedies to consider:-

Arsenicum   There are severe anorexic tendencies, always feeling cold, too neat and usually exhausted. A loner, worse for company or any close contact.

Natrum mur   Tearful depression with tension and anxiety are the key features, with severe weight loss and lack of interest in food. He is often worse for sea air, contact with others, never fully at ease in their company.

Pulsatilla   The anorexia is severe but varied, worse in summer and for heat, improved by both company and attention. Mood swings are a feature from laughter to irritability or tears.There is low self-esteem, and the body imagery is often distorted.

Silicea   Weakness is a feature, lacking drive and confidence. He tends to sweat on covered areas of the body (e.g. the head or arm-pit).

Tuberculinum   There is severe weight loss, pallor, and exhaustion, a tendency to a recurrent dry chesty cough. Always better for travel.

ANXIETY

Anxiety is a feeling of anguish, a sense of discomfort or malaise, an indescribable feeling of vague apprehension in the pit of the stomach due to tension and fear. It is often felt in the head or chest, across the shoulders, sometimes as restless tension within the arms or legs, sweating and pale with apprehension and dread. Aggression and short-fuse irritability also occurs with intolerant attitudes and dislike of change. Even holidays are seen as unnecessary, a demand and drain on energy as well as financial resources. All anxiety is a form of fear; taking flight from a difficulty, or an imagined one, despite an underlying wish to face up to the situation and not to feel a coward or a failure. There is a lack of confidence, coupled with an intense anticipation of disaster or failure, leading to humiliation, loss of love, support and affection.

For many, anxiety is a long-standing problem, a way of life - really a refuge from it. Often previous attempts at treatment have ended in only a partial improvement or failure with resumption of the old anxiety patterns. This demonstrates the power and intensity of the underlying neurotic drive, and its determination to survive and persist with old personality patterns, despite the most skilled of interventions. Symptoms may occur in a perfectly familiar social situation, even one planned and looked forward to. Overall attitudes are often more important than the actual symptoms, with complaints of chronic fatigue, lack of drive or energy after the least effort, and nothing is ever really right; enjoyed or worthy of enthusiasm. Life seems just one problem after another as pessimism and complaining reluctance asserts itself in any social or new situation when there

35

is a change of routine. Symptoms often seem entirely illogical. The friends are often known and well-liked, yet it seems that every emotion only leads downward into a spiral of excited anticipation mixed with fear and foreboding, feeling unable to cope and wanting to run away or hide. Other people are often both liked and avoided, seen as a threat, or their success is felt to imply failure. At the same time, there is always loneliness and a longing for real contact and closeness, to be able to give out and receive greater affection.

Character traits which aggravate the condition
There is a tendency to create disasters out of change and challenge, with a rigid, narrow negative approach to life and problems giving a perspective of potential failure and creating fear. Any form of failure is seen as a total devastation and disaster, leading to loss of love and rejection. There is a tendency to go over past hurts and difficulties repeatedly, reinforcing memories of pain and aggravating anxiety.

Practical steps to improve things
Try to see each evolving moment more positively, leading to new chances, challenges and opportunities. Allow each new situation to emerge fully without pre-judging, changing it, or expecting a disaster. Try to remain much more you with others, not intimidating yourself. If you feel depressed, frightened or angry, accept this as something reflecting **you**, as you are now, not a failure or something negative. See life more as a journey, each stopping place or encounter, a challenge, a way of learning, maturing, a new experience gained. Think less negatively and less destructively. Aim to be natural and yourself as life unfolds.

Remedies to consider:-

Aconitum   A remedy for acute stress anxiety, linked to fear or shock with agitation.

Arnica   There is a bruised numb sense of anxiety, often caused by a recent shock or trauma.

Arsenicum   For restless anxiety with depression, fear and anguish. All symptoms are worse at night. Obsessional neatness and control are a feature.

Lycopodium   A remedy for anticipatory anxiety with insecurity. Pseudo-maturity and impatience, are characteristic.

Natrum mur   There is severe anxiety associated with tearful depression and fatigue.

Pulsatilla   The symptoms of fear and lack of confidence are variable and often dramatic. Tearful emotional mood-swings are common. There is intolerance of heat.

Sepia   For anxiety with a heavy dragging down sense of fatigue and irritability. Indifference to others.

ASSERTIVENESS-LOW

This is usually a long-standing character attitude. There is a tendency to hold back opinions, feelings, spontaneity, in any social or work situation, especially where there is a difference of opinion, a challenge, disagreement, disapproval or argument. There is nearly always a problem of low self-esteem and self-criticism often a way of avoiding making a definite statement, or having a position on anything which is controversial. The problem is frequently learned and encouraged in childhood by parents or grandparents who support conformity, being diplomatic, and never taking up or expressing anything controversial. A non-questioning non-challenging, withholding approach to life was often rewarded as 'good' behaviour. This was because the parents did not know how to respond, or they had also been brought up to avoid dissent, never to challenge or disagree because they felt threatened or embarrassed. As a child there may have been acts of aggression, bullying, physical abuse and violence. This may have been from a parent and often alcohol-related, sometimes from a teacher or older sibling. There may have been bullying from another child which terrorised the child. The trauma may have fixated the character into attitudes of withdrawal and passivity which blocked further creative growth and to some extent limited achievement and experience.

Some degree of independence and rebellion are both essential for the healthy growth of the child, and later the adolescent, to break away from the yoke of the parents and childish attitudes. To make this break, healthy assertiveness is essential for everyone.

Where assertiveness is low, the individual has usually learned that to take flight into low-profile behaviour is safer than confronting a particular problem. This is then carried on into adult life. There may be reluctance to be firm or certain about anything; even to have an opinion, to be assertive, to agree or disagree, because of anxiety. It is easy to develop attitudes of keeping feelings inside, because of fear of criticism, dislike of argument, and a vague fear of not knowing how to cope with what others might demand or expect. Fear of being on view, seen as foolish and laughed at, can be a further aspect of the problem which weakens self-assertiveness. Anxiety about losing control is often a factor, especially where strong feelings of anger, hurt, resentment and rage have been kept locked away inside, closely allied to need, loneliness and overwhelming love.

Character traits which aggravate the condition

There is a tendency to withdraw from the direct spontaneous expression of thoughts and feelings, often from fear of punishment and disapproval. Shyness, keeping other people at a distance, hiding true needs and feelings, always remote, creates fear. Passivity and over-dependent attitudes cause further weakness.

Practical steps to improve things

Practise saying 'No' more often, and expressing disagreement. Try to say what you think and feel in every situation, to be more you. Others may be a little surprised initially, but will respect you more. Tell them what you are doing and why, but don't over-emphasise the changes or agree just for the sake of it. Take time out to clarify what you really feel about people of every age, position and status, and practise being more open and positive with them. Start slowly, but be consistent.

Remedies to consider:-

Arsenicum   Meaningful contact with others is either avoided or kept strictly at a distance. Obsessional neatness and rigid attitudes are a feature.

Aurum met   There is withdrawal from others because of a self-critical depressive mood.

Lycopodium   An overall lack of confidence exists, often hidden under a facade of maturity.

Natrum mur   The problem is mainly related to lack of confidence and malaise in all social situations.

Phosphorus   Confidence is low and there is a constant need for reassurance and acceptance.

Pulsatilla   Shyness, withdrawal, lack of self-confidence, fear of aggression or disagreement, passivity, are daily barriers to healthy assertiveness.

Silicea   Fear, insecurity, lack of self-confidence and drive, all combine to limit assertiveness.

ASTHMA

Asthma is associated with a nervous, highly strung, sensitive, artistic temperament, reacting to pressures or stress with tightness of the chest. It often starts in childhood, at any time after weaning, related to a food or milk allergy. It is also common in adults with no childhood history of chest problems.

Several factors seem to play a role in the chest sensitivity. The illness tends to run in families, and it is common for one parent to have been asthmatic or 'chesty' at some time, or there is a history of chest problems in at least one member of the family. In many asthmatics there has been at least one previous severe chest infection, such as pneumonia, which has sensitized the chest and weakened it. It may have also frightened the child because of the intense emotional and fear reactions of the family at that time.

Asthma is often related to stress, getting nervous or over-excited, anxious about challenges, social events, and often never really comfortable or at ease with others. It may be provoked by anticipation, particularly before an examination, interview, a new job or school.

Some asthmatics appear to show no obvious signs of a stress link and even the suggestion of a possible psychological connection is fiercely denied or resented by the sufferer or his family. They deny any form of psychological tension, forcing all critical or negative feelings deeply into the psyche with a facade of happiness and the absence of any worries. This form of social denial within the family is itself a major stress, difficult if not impossible to live with and live up to.

In families of this type, any form of adverse emotion is ruled out and it is common to find other persistent forms of psychosomatic illness, such as migraine or colitis, blood-pressure, or indigestion problems.

In most asthmatics, there is a combination of physical and psychological causes, a tendency to over-react to any emotional situation. Any move away from routine and the usual patterns, causes a lowering of vitality and resistance with heightened tension. An asthma reaction may be provoked by almost any adverse physical circumstances. These then act as triggers - typically exposure to moulds or pollens, animal hair, a viral common cold, a drop in barometric pressure or temperature, or an increase in humidity levels.

Character traits which aggravate the conditions
There is a tendency to be over-sensitive, lacking confidence, fearing disapproval and worrying too much about what others think. There is often fear of expressing any anger or resentment, because of conformist character traits.

Practical steps to improve things
Relax much more and build up fitness by regular physical exercise and a healthy diet. Regular walking or swimming is ideal, but it should be regular, at least three times weekly. Slowly increase the time and distance, depending upon your age and fitness. Use an exercise cycle during the winter months. Try to remain calm in pressure situations, keeping the chest relaxed and free from tension. At all times stay in touch with your feelings and allow them to be expressed openly. Be more spontaneous with your emotions. Practise regular deep relaxation or meditation.

Remedies to consider:-

Antimon. tart   Dizziness, fatigue and vague confusion are the main stress symptoms together with the asthma.

Arsenicum   Fussy, obsessional mannerisms and avoidance of others, the asthma worse after midnight.

Dulcamara   There is anxiety about the future, also restlessness, with impatient, irritable moods. The asthma is worse on waking and from cold or damp air.

Ignatia   The asthma is associated with grief, mourning and loss, with marked depression and loss of drive or energy.

Ipecacuanha   Irritability is marked, the chest wheezy with a moist loose cough. Persistent nausea is often a feature.

Kali carb   Exhaustion with anxiety is present, all symptoms worse in the early night hours, between 3-5.00 a.m.

Lachesis   All chest symptoms are worse after sleep. The mood is variable, often anxious or suspicious. Over-talkative, and intolerant of tight clothing.

Lycopodium   All symptoms are worse in the late afternoon and early evening between 4-8.00 p.m. Lack of confidence, and also constantly seeking for attention and reassurance.

Medorrhinum   Tearful, moody and depressed, often impatient. Time seems to drag endlessly, the asthma better for sea or moist air, and lying on the stomach.

Phosphorus   Anxiety with fear and tension. Over-sensitive, all symptoms are worse from heat, or changes of barometric pressure.

Psorinum   He is chilly at the height of summer, at times despairing and anxious in mood. The asthma is worse from cold air or draughts.

BACKACHE

This is one of the commonest symptoms of stress and tension, often the first area to feel the strain from underlying pressure, frustration or loss of confidence.

Many adults find themselves trapped in a job or a relationship where they feel anger and frustration, and are not able to fully express themselves. Sometimes they feel insufficiently valued. Unless such feelings are discussed and dealt with in an open positive way, their negative energy can seep into the skeletal muscular system undermining ease of movement and posture and causing discomfort or spasm. This may first appear as severe low back pain which may be incapacitating for weeks or months, and only relieved by complete bed rest. The underlying cause of the problem is often due to a combination of months of stress tension and frustration, combined with a poor posture.

Any activity, even driving the car, walking, or bending down movements tend to be rushed, badly timed, or jerky, quick and precipitant, not relaxed, paced, flowing, smooth or harmonious. The combination of underlying tension with hours of sitting in a poor spinal position, often in a chair which is not ergometric and designed to support the spine correctly, causes a chronic low back situation, this may be associated with ligament strain and sometimes misalignment of one of the lower vertebrae. If the spine is not in its correct position, it should be adjusted by an osteopath or chiropractor before beginning homoeopathic treatment. Regular relaxation and massage are also beneficial and recommended when recurrent stress backache is a problem.

Character traits which aggravate the condition

There is a tendency to retain feelings of indignation, irritability and resentment. Such feelings are pushed down, at the same time as over-reacting to every demand and situation:- over-competitive, too intense, never sufficiently relaxed, impatient, precipitate. You may also allow yourself to get too easily rattled and under pressure, at the same time quickly getting rid of the feelings, making everything rushed and impulsive, pushing tension down into the spine or low-back region.

Practical steps to improve things

If you feel pressurised or stressed, don't allow it to build-up. Either get out of the pressure situation for a time, taking a quiet walk, time out to think more clearly, or if this is not possible, practise letting go, being more open and frank whenever you feel a pressure situation starting to build up. Avoid excessive competitive situations until you are more relaxed and try to prevent tension building up. Don't struggle to be best or Mr Perfect, just be yourself, appreciate others, in this way also enjoying yourself more.

If you feel yourself getting tense, keep your spine and neck straight (but not tight or rigid). Avoid clasping your shoulders forward to bury yourself in your chest (perhaps to hide there), as this will put a great deal of strain and tension on your low back and worsen any existing problems.

Remedies to consider:-

Aconitum   For acute backache associated
                with fear and agitation.

Agaricus   There is painful stiffness along the
                whole of the spine, worse for
                bending and sensitive to touch.

Arnica   The pain is of a bruised type and
                often linked to emotional shock,
                strain, or following an accident.

Berberis   For burning lumbar back pain and
                stiffness. The pain may spread to
                involve the nearby abdominal
                area, bladder, or the groin.

Ignatia   A remedy for backache following
                an acute loss, grief, or mourning
                reaction.

Natrum mur For backache caused by acute
                emotional tension, improved by
                firm local pressure.

Nux vomica For low back pain associated with
                tension, spasm, and irritability.
                Constipation is often a problem.

Radium brom For painful low back problems
                associated with tension, fatigue
                and irritability.

BLOOD-PRESSURE

Obesity, diet, and stress are major factors producing a rise in blood-pressure, but it is often also linked to psychological insecurity. Stress and tension cause exhaustion and fatigue, often a compelling hunger with a strong compulsion to eat high calorie snack foods which lead to an increase in weight. The spilling over of tension and stifled emotion into the cardiovascular system provokes the increased blood-pressure and consequently greater work for the heart. Any increase in pressure, also causes increased wear and tear of the arterial walls and an increased tendency for arteriosclerosis or hardening of the arteries.

Repressed emotional energy may act directly on the circulatory system, with a greater stroke volume (pump action) of the heart, leading to palpitations, or chest fullness and awareness of the heart's actions. There may also be extra beats with heart irregularity, sometimes a racing pulse (paroxysmal tachycardia), flushing, or sweating, as the pores of the skin dilate from the heat produced from dilated vessels just under the skin. Adrenalin is poured out at the slightest emotional challenge or fear situation, anticipating an aggressive or a flight response and causing a temporary rise in blood-pressure. If this is constantly repeated, levels may become permanently raised.

Over-intense, excessive, competitive relationships are often the underlying problem, combined with inability to express anger, rage and frustration. The body acts as if it is constantly going to fight, producing an out-flowing of energy and using up reserves with a raised blood-pressure.

Character traits which aggravate the condition

Often the major problem is bottling-up feelings, especially anger or resentment, not appreciating that this is damaging. The freeing of such feelings is essential for changes to occur. There is a tendency to be too controlled, often over long periods, building-up emotions like a pressure cooker without a safety valve and exploding in an uncontrollable surge of feelings which push up the blood-pressure. There is a tendency to be far too easily irritated, which is also a reason for high readings.

Practical steps to improve things

Lose weight **slowly** over a period of weeks or months, bringing it down to target levels for your age and height. Preferably do this by developing sensible eating habits which you can maintain. Don't try to lose weight by dieting, as it is likely to be short term and to fail. Eat sensibly, avoiding salt, excessive amounts of dairy products and red meat. Take garlic daily, either fresh, or as a supplement. Avoid heavy work and lifting, especially in heat. Exercise regularly, but gently and at first, never to excess. Relax or meditate, for at least 10-15 minutes daily, and practise this in any situation of tension.

When driving, try to relax, especially if you find yourself gripping the wheel, allowing the arms and legs to release any strain. Always allow feelings to come up and be expressed as they emerge, without swift or self-denigratory judgment. Try to be less self-critical and less critical of others. Beginning from the moment you wake in the morning, find a natural rhythm for everything in life, trying to stay in an easy, smooth rhythmic attitude throughout the day.

Remedies to consider:-

Aconitum   For acute problems associated with fear and agitation.

Aurum met   There are violent palpitations, worse for exercise. Irregular beatings of the heart occur, with a sense of anguish in the heart region.

Digitalis   The heart beat is irregular with extra beats followed by a pause, the pulse thready and slow.

Natrum mur   Depression, anxiety, avoidance of others, exhaustion and tearfulness are marked. All symptoms are worse for sea air.

Pulsatilla   There are variable symptoms but always worse from heat. Tearfulness is common and there is a tendency to be dramatic.

Spartium   A useful remedy which slows the heart down and reduces blood-pressure.

Spigelia   A remedy for violent palpitations, worse for bending forwards, and in the morning. The heart feels oppressed causing a sense of anguish.

BLUSHING

Blushing is an important aspect of shyness and a very common problem, particularly during adolescence. It occurs at a time when pride is strong and emotions run high. The least suggestion of criticism, feeling vulnerable, or hurt, is felt with burning passion and resentment. As with blood-pressure problems, the emotional tension is reflected through the circulatory system, the facial blood vessels becoming dilated, the skin hot and sweating, the cheek area reddened.

This is a particularly embarrassing problem because it is feared that others will notice any discomfort or comment on it, in order to provoke laughter or humiliation. Blushing can occur at any age, when confidence is weak or lost. It is particularly associated with problems of self-consciousness, dealing with authority (parental) figures and linked to sexual preoccupations, often because of fear of sexual difficulties. Guilt feelings are linked to an intensive self-awareness and shame which creates the circulatory stimulus to flush up. There are usually many mixed emotions, associated with a strong desire for attention and to be noticed.

The condition improves with maturity. Homoeopathy helps the problem to be resolved by bringing any underlying conflicts to consciousness, where they can more easily be dealt with. It also acts as a stimulus to greater psychological maturity and balance.

Character traits which aggravate the condition

Passivity is one of the major attitudes which causes the difficulties, also problems handling aggression, because of fear of loss of control. There is a tendency to feel weak or inadequate because of endless comparisons with other people. Building them up as superior in some way in order to push yourself down and feel less successful, adds to the problems. There is failure to see yourself as an individual, different rather than inferior, and at a different point on the road to self-knowledge and maturity.

Practical steps to improve things

Don't attempt to hide or deny the particular problem area or even the embarrassment. Accept this as your particular weak or problem area at the moment, and that it is not something to feel ashamed about. See the blushing as something you are working on which will evolve and change. It is important to acknowledge that everyone has some areas of weakness or problem and that your blushing does not in any way diminish you or imply inferiority or failure. Don't feel ashamed of the blushing, but accept it as something that thousands of others feel and experience and try to find a way to use it creatively rather than in a destructive way. See blushing as your individual way of expressing a conflict. If you try to keep the intensity of your feelings, or the blushing hidden and secret, this will only worsen it. Practise accepting yourself more, and at the same time remain easy and relaxed. If you find yourself blushing, try making a comment about it, or even a joke, drawing attention to it, rather than the opposite. Psychologically this will give you much more control over the blushing, rather than it controlling you, and this will help it to diminish.

Remedies to consider:-

Baryta carb   There is dejection, vagueness and lack of drive, with inability to take decisions. A tendency to be tearful and forgetful.

Belladonna   For acute problems with a red face, sweating, agitation, and often states of severe anxiety and fear, worse for jolting or draughts of cold air.

Carbo veg   Any anxiety is worse in the evening, with a slow flow of ideas or feeling tearful. Indigestion with flatulence, occurs in the upper stomach region.

Phosphorus   There is extreme sensitivity and restless anxiety, constantly seeking reassurance and acceptance.

Pulsatilla   For variable symptoms of shyness and a tearful lack of confidence. All symptoms are worse for heat and any new social situation. There is an absence of thirst.

Sulphur   All the shyness symptoms are rather variable and untidy, associated with frequent gassy intestinal upsets and chronic skin problems.

COLITIS

Colitis occurs when stress problems are referred to the intestine or colon. The commonest symptoms are an irritable bowel, with frequent soft or watery stools, pain, flatulence, wind and spasm, sometimes passing mucus and blood.

The underlying temperament tends to be rigid, far too controlled, and a perfectionist, over-intense, often competitive, driven by deadlines, rules and ambitions. This leaves little time to rest and relax, pause or think more imaginatively and creatively, because of the underlying drives and pressures.

Anxiety and fear often run at a high level because of an inability to ever fully relax, creating tense, uneasy relationships with others. The colitis subject may never feel fully natural or at ease with others, constantly on guard and mindful of being dominated, made to feel small or inadequate. There is often a sense of panic, wanting to rush out of an unfamiliar social situation because of not knowing what to say, or how to react.

Colitis can be an acute problem, of short-duration, only occurring over a period of days or weeks. But it can also be intermittent, with long periods - often months or years without symptoms and between attacks. It may also become chronic, with a persistent watery diarrhoea and jelly-like mucus or blood on the stools.

If severe, the bowel may ulcerate, become infected, develop painful, enlarged lymphatic glands in the colon area and require surgical resection (removal), particularly if there is an ulcerated or narrowed area.

Character traits which aggravate the condition

There is a tendency to allow irritability and resentment to build-up and accumulate, but rarely expressed directly. The direct more open expression of all emotions is controlled, distorted and suppressed. Verbal discussion is also kept minimal when it concerns feelings, and all emotion tends to be held in and pushed down.

Practical steps to improve things

Aim to be much more open and spontaneous, expressing your feelings and ideas as you experience them. Share more of yourself and be more open. If you feel angry, say so, but be less controlled and don't seek to be perfect. Also try to be more outgoing, and even 'untidy' with your emotions, as long as the feelings expressed are spontaneous and really reflect **you** as you are feeling right now. Avoid allowing resentment to fester or accumulate and get all your feelings out into the open as soon as you know they are there, even before if possible. At the same time stay calm and cool as you do so.

Remedies to consider:-

Agaricus For griping abdominal pain, worse in the morning with rumbling noises and distention, also diarrhoea with flatus.

Ammonium mur There is griping pain, with flatulence and wind and a burning soreness. All symptoms are better for local pressure.

Magnesium phos A useful remedy for colitis with severe colicky pains.

Natrum sulph For windy, colicky morning diarrhoea, sensitive to the least change in the weather. Symptoms are worse for cold or damp.

Podophyllum There is a painless watery diarrhoea with mucus.

Sulphur Indicated for offensive morning diarrhoea with windy flatulence. The skin is often infected and all symptoms are worse for heat or contact with water.

Thuja There is a combination of colicky pains and windy flatulence, as if something is 'alive' and moving in the abdomen. All symptoms are worse for damp, and from coffee.

COMPETITIVENESS

The need to win and be best at everything at all costs places enormous pressure on the individual. It differs from a more healthy attitude of trying to win in order to give of your best in a game or sport. The healthier emphasis is on performance, breaking through barriers and limitations, seeking challenges to extend the self, but not just the winning or beating the other person. Excessive competitiveness can enter into every aspect of life, into every encounter. This is because there is a need to prove that no other person is better at anything, you are trying to do, because this is seen as a failure and leads to inferiority feelings.

Frequently the unconscious drive is to impress a parent, to do better than a sibling who as a child was felt to gain more attention and love from the parents by being older, quicker, smarter, better looking or faster. The attitudes of the mother or father may have caused the problem, only really impressed, (rewarding the child with a physical hug), when he was top or came first at something. In this way they unconsciously reinforced feelings that he must of necessity always be a'winner' in order to gain affection and approval.

The father himself may have been very competitive in his own attitudes, and felt to only understand and respond to this kind of behaviour.

Ultimately excessive competitiveness must fail because of the pressures it imposes, and it is impossible to sustain. Under the surface, there is a dread of failure in any form, because this means being unacceptable and unlovable, often causing irritability and depression.

Character traits which aggravate the condition

There is an inability to accept failure or anything other than best, with intolerance of a mistake, an error, or not being best and favourite all the time. Pressure occurs because of over-demanding attitudes, pushing, driving the self to limits all the time and never adequately resting. The individual may be even competitive when talking and rarely listens to what others have to say. The deep insecurity problems are also not usually acknowledged.

Practical steps to improve things

Try to play for the sake of playing, to talk easily for the sake of talking and giving, not always seeking to be best or to score points over others. Realise that you do not have to always win at everything, or always be best, liked, or even loved all the time. Try a more 'take it or leave it' attitude. Don't strive for an impression, just be yourself, natural and calm. Practise losing gracefully. Enjoy the game more, and the dialogue. Don't only see life as a contest you have to win. Try to sense what fundamentally matters, gives you most pleasure, confidence and a sense of identity. It is often just simple things, the time you spend with others, or being yourself, not having to be a winner all the time. Spend more time enjoying others, more relaxed and stop trying to be best (really the favourite child) all the time.

Remedies to consider:-

Chamomilla
There is anxiety and groaning, restlessness when he does not get his own way or win all the time. Often irritable and impatient.

Nux vomica
The whole approach to life is far too intense and zealous. Every action is carried to an extreme and is competitive, with deadlines and pressures imposed on the self and others, most of which are unnecessary. There is also failure to delegate. A useful remedy for the irritable stressed executive, when everything is carried out to excess.

Phosphorus
Much of the competition is for attention and reassurance. Almost every encounter is tense and emotional, causing flushing up with excitement, anxiety, pressure and over-sensitivity.

Platinum
There is a tendency to be arrogant and proud, looking down on others. He is often quarrelsome with tears, or in a fearful mood.

Staphysagria
The competition is impulsive, irritable, and often violent or resentful.

COMPULSIVE BEHAVIOUR

This includes any form of compulsive, repetitive, or excessive behaviour, where there is lack of reasonable control. Some typical examples are compulsive:- eating, gambling, alcohol intake, dieting, spending, smoking, deviant sexual behaviour:- for example, voyeurism, indecent exposure, a preoccupation with pornographic magazines or videos.

There may be a tendency to repeat negative patterns of behaviour such as spending to excess on food, buying clothes which are not essential and which cannot really be afforded. Often beneath a compulsion lie feelings of deep depression or deprivation and the only way to feel better for a short time is to go out and spend some money. Giving to oneself - buying clothes, furniture, food, is always pleasurable to some degree, but when it becomes compulsive and out of control, it becomes a stress because it is excessive and inappropriate. At times, giving in to a compulsive habit or drive, seems the only thing in life which brings relief from tension or a mood of despair.

Compulsive eating is a problem which increases depression. Inevitably there is a weight gain, leading to either mild or severe obesity, adding to underlying problems of guilt feelings, often dislike of self, causing a greater tendency to binge in order to feel better.

Compulsive gambling is a social illness where excitement and risk are craved in order to give a temporary respite from problem areas which are not being constructively dealt with.

Unless it is mild, the compulsive pattern is eventually self-defeating and leads to frustration, feelings of failure, and often tension. Compulsive behaviour is often an attempt to drive away the need for a fundamental change of attitudes, aims, and life-style. Underlying depression, fear, and lack of confidence, may impede the changes necessary to bring this into reality.

Character traits which aggravate the condition

Control is the main feature in this type of personality, with a marked limitation of spontaneity in all aspects and often controlling others. All forms of open and free self-expression are severely limited by routine, rituals, strict adherence to order, and predictable responses.

Practical steps to improve things

Aim to break out from your defensive patterns of order and ritual by deliberately neglecting to follow what the compulsive patterns are attempting to repeat and impose. You may find this difficult and slow at first, but start by neglecting any daily chores which have become an obsessional ritual, rather than a task to be completed. Also try being less of a perfectionist, less critical of others and more out-going and generous towards them. Keep a close eye open for any rigid patterns, and try to find different ways of breaking out of these, at the same time avoid creating new ones. Always aim for greater spontaneity, ease of self-expression and relaxation, not pre-judging others or the issues which really concern you. If stopping a compulsive habit causes anxiety, temporarily increase the dosage and frequency of the homoeopathic potency you are taking. Practise regular periods of deep relaxation or meditation.

Remedies to consider:-

Arsenicum   For anguish and despair, all symptoms worse in the early night hours. He is over-sensitive and frequently depressed.

Calcarea   There is lack of vital energy and body heat. The body is usually chilly, covered in sweat and overweight. Anxiety and fear are marked, with frequent nervous or compulsive movements of an obsessional type.

Nux vomica   The temperament is compulsive in attitudes, with an over-zealous, intense, irritable approach to life and others. Confidence is often supreme, alternating between bouts of depression and brooding revenge fantasies.

Sulphur   There is a compulsive tendency to be idealistic, to philosophise, repeat himself, often in an attempt to boost flagging self-confidence or to gain an audience and support. But most of the talk is vague and speculative with little real drive or substance to it. Irritability and depression are common, with chronic bowel and skin problems and intolerance of heat.

CONCENTRATION-POOR

This may be due to either physical or emotional factors, but any form of stress is likely to undermine concentration because it drains energy and reserves. Pollution, noise, vibration, poor air quality, poor quality of light, also interfere with the reception and processing of incoming stimuli within the brain and are a common cause of impaired concentration.

Emotional factors divert energy and attention away from concentration because energy is taken up with the particular problem, the body giving biological priority to stress pressures because they are often expressed physically, or experienced as an acute crisis and a basic survival issue. Any emotional problem which cannot be immediately solved reduces focusing and attention in all areas, including work, until it is resolved.

Character traits which aggravate the condition
A tendency to be always thinking of other things, rushing ahead, rather than staying with the matters in hand. Often the mind is overloaded, leading to fatigue and memory lapses. Fear and anxiety undermine concentration, and drain drive or energy.

Practical steps to improve things
Avoid making lists, and keep the mind on one thing at a time until each project is completed. Try to link ideas you wish to recall with specific situations. Broaden your interests into new areas, and develop new skills. Relax as much as possible and consider meditating. Avoid anticipating problems, or thinking in advance that you cannot complete or resolve a particular problem.

Remedies to consider:-

Aconitum   There is a situation of acute fear or emotional shock, with restless anxiety, often agitation.

Gelsemium   Apathy, anxiety, lack of self-confidence, fear of others, or any new situation undermines concentration levels.

Ignatia   The difficulty is related to a highly painful situation of grief, loss, or mourning.

Lycopodium   Concentration is impaired by a 'butterfly mentality', constantly distracted by thoughts and ideas running ahead of the matter in hand. Lack of confidence causes attention-seeking behaviour.

Natrum mur   The lack of concentration is due to severe emotional stress problems with a tearful depression, fatigue, lack of energy and drive.

Nux vomica   Irritability is marked, the mind over-zealous and far too intense to take in new thoughts or ideas.

Sepia   There is a combination of irritability, fatigue, and indifference to others.

CONFIDENCE LOSS

This is a common problem, as it severely limits many important areas of contact with others, particularly ease and freedom of self-expression, and relationships with others. There is a tendency to feel under pressure, inadequate in some way, or not living up to expectations. Criticism and often anger are usually turned against the self, finding fault with almost any form of personal expression or encounter, self-accusing and 'nit-picking' over the most ordinary everyday matters. Perfectionist attitudes can be very undermining and intolerant, as if to say, 'You are a nuisance, always doing the wrong thing at the wrong time time'.

There is also a tendency to be short on patience with others, not 'suffering fools gladly', and making insufficient allowances for others. These hypercritical attitudes cause unpopularity, becoming alienated and adds to the misery of being without real friends. Whatever is done, seems to end in disaster, adding to lack of confidence, because of a weakening of social contacts.

Some of the most common causes of confidence loss are simple and obvious - the breakdown of a marriage or a relationship, a divorce, loss of a job, failing an examination or an interview, a sudden unexpected illness or accident, or following an operation which led to a period of complete dependency and incapacity, having to give up the controls for a time.

The confidence loss may have always been present in some degree since childhood, and it is not easy to positively define the causes or to find an answer.

In many cases, the origins of the problem lie within the family and the type of upbringing. Some of the most common are:- an over-anxious taxing parent, mental or physical illness of a parent with long periods away from home for treatment followed by drugs which blunted affection and sensitivity. There is often lack of communication within the family, over-strict rigid attitudes, intolerance, especially during childhood or adolescence, and frequently about sexual matters such as the onset of menstruation. Unhappy experiences at day or boarding school, the premature loading of a young child with adult personal problems, including their problems and attitudes towards the opposite sex, are other stress factors which undermine confidence.

Character traits which aggravate the condition

There is a tendency to be too self-critical, to denigrate achievements and to over-value others. This may lead to problems of envy and jealousy, or excessive attention-seeking behaviour, sometimes expressed in a negative way as feelings of inferiority. These are often the reverse of unconscious feelings, but ensure that a critical, aggressive or competitive response is never expressed overtly, except through tears.

Practical steps to improve things

Avoid judging what you or others do or say. Just do your best for today and enjoy it. Express yourself to the full as naturally as possible, but avoid damaging self-criticism or negating yourself in any way. Try also to avoid idealising others, because this puts them on a pedestal (safe from criticism or retaliation), but too remote for you to relate to. Just be yourself, evolve and develop without imposing blocks, or limitations.

Remedies to consider:-

Arnica The underlying personality is damaged or psychologically bruised, because of a previous hurt, loss, or rejection, causing confidence loss.

Causticum There is an anxious, fearful state of mind, apprehensive of change and quickly feeling exhausted.

Cicuta virosa Early morning anxiety is marked. Oversensitive, and can quickly become tearful or depressed.

Ignatia The problem is linked to grief and loss, usually associated with tearful depression and anguish.

Lycopodium The whole personality make-up is too much in a hurry, everything rushed and precipitate. He is always anxious to please. This may lead to pseudo-maturity.

Pulsatilla Shyness, fear of disapproval, or rejection, wanting to please, a shy tearful disposition, tends to undermine all confidence.

Silicea There is lack of drive and energy, needing constant support and encouragement. Weakness, with a tendency to run from challenges.

DEPRESSION

This is one of the most important stress problem areas and to some degree, almost invariably present. It may vary in intensity, appearing as critical irritable moods or threats, or a cold seemingly calculated withdrawal and rejection, when things don't go as planned, or there is a difficulty or hitch in plans. A lowering or flattening of mood is common, everything 'piano' and subdued. Often a 'down' mood occurs for no obvious reason, it just seems to occur on waking, not feeling like company, wanting to be left alone, reluctant to talk, share ideas and feelings, to retire, perhaps sulk alone, sorry for yourself and convinced that no one really cares or understands. Of course this makes no sense, especially when the depressive mood has led to a withdrawal of affection and approval because you are feeling annoyed and irritated - usually with yourself and don't want to admit why. Depression may also emerge as a drink problem, a combination of short-fuse anger and irritability, fed by the alcohol intake. Sometimes it presents in a more physical way, as chronic indigestion, long-standing problems which are never fully diagnosed, an incapacitating low back problem, or a joint problem which grumbles on and no amount of treatment resolves or improves it. There is often a plethora of complaining misery, putting up with suffering in a martyr-like way coupled with a 'nobody really cares' attitude. Self-pity and lack of humour adds to the load carried and the 'down' in mood.

Stress depression does not usually constitute an illness as such, but it is important to relieve the condition in order to prevent an undermining of communication and social isolation which may impinge upon others fuelling guilt or irritation. Friends and family often feel defeated and useless, helpless to do or say anything that will relieve the suffering. Almost anything said to cause comfort, or a more balanced viewpoint, is derided or belittled, and all attempts to intervene or help, seem to make matters worse. The family may eventually feel defeated and depressed. It is often at this point, that the depression starts to lift, the mood changes, there is a better feeling and suddenly again there is light at the end of the tunnel.

Character traits which aggravate the condition

There is a tendency to push down and deny all disappointment and conflict and not to openly express feelings of love, need, anger, missing, hurt. Such feelings are more directed inwards, at the self, always taking the blame, keeping conflict under a stiff upper lip, not admitting the destructive nature of any hurt. This denial (often due to pride), is destructive to personality development and freedom of expression.

Practical steps to improve things

Keep all feelings, both positive and negative, out in the open, as soon as you are aware of them. You can always apologise later, if you feel you have exaggerated in your opinions and attitudes, but a social 'faux pas' is less likely to be damaging and to lead to a crisis. Be realistic in your expectations of others and don't idealise them. If you are feeling down, don't analyse or even try to think too much, just be at ease, staying close to people you like and are in touch with. Keep physically fit and exercise to counter any tendency to narrow rigid thinking. Try not to think obsessionally, or to be taken over by what might have happened or been said. Aim to be more flexible.

Remedies to consider:-

Aurum met   For more despairing depression, often associated with palpitations and painful joint problems.

Capsicum   He is preoccupied with the past, homesick, and always feels threatened by change.

Ignatia   There is a hysterical make-up, and a tendency to over-react, usually related to grief and loss.

Lycopodium   There is a sense of apprehension, depression due to insecurity, and a dislike of being alone in the house. Self-confidence is low.

Natrum mur   Stress-related depression is worse for sympathy or social contacts. Irritable and easily tearful, worse for sea air, music, and heat.

Sepia   Feels dragged down by pressures, exhaustion, and depression. Irritability is marked. There is often indifference to loved ones. All symptoms are worse before a thunder storm, and better once tears are shed, also improved by dancing.

DIVORCE

In our pressurised society, divorce is one of the major social symptoms of stress. About one marriage in two now ends in divorce (1992 statistics) and many are opting for the less demanding commitments of a common law association. Every divorce is painful in some way, felt to be a loss and a failure, and often associated with profound feelings of guilt.

Each divorce is a breaking of close ties, former hopes and aspirations, an ending of a chapter, and the beginning of another. But however bright the future, a new relationship waiting in the wings, or already embarked upon, the pain and scars of divorce have a tendency to run deep and may cause future problems. Children need especial consideration and understanding, seen regularly, kept informed and reassured, to keep damage minimal. There may be acrimonious disputes about custody, maintenance, or access to the children, creating additional hurt, putting future trust and confidence at risk; especially if the divorce is lengthy.

Depression and stress problems are particularly likely to surface at this time because of the insecurity and uncertainty caused. To some extent, every divorced person feels abandoned, betrayed, and let down, promoting feelings of anger and frustration. It is difficult, because of past attachments, to totally forget the past, and even with a trusted new partner it is possible to feel frightened of making a commitment. Sleep problems, fear of being alone in the house, depression, overeating in order to compensate for loneliness and frustration may cause a weight problem and add further to feelings of gloom.

After any divorce it is essential to allow plenty of time with a new partner to develop open sharing and communication. The high failure rate of second marriages and subsequent relationships is often because of the depth of the hurt, loss of confidence and trust (in the self as well as of others). This is often not understood and sufficient priority made for it. A second divorce may not be as traumatic as the first, because there has not been the same degree of commitment and attachment given to a first marriage. Nevertheless it is a further hurt and adds to any tendency to remain 'safe' and distant, and (in theory at least), less vulnerable.

Character traits which aggravate the condition
There are often rigid resentful attitudes, causing a more difficult, 'messy' divorce. Lack of confidence may create fears which are inappropriate to the real problems. Sometimes there is a tendency to cling to a relationship which has virtually ended, yet denying the inevitability of break-up and divorce.

Positive steps to improve things
Be open and more generous towards your ex-partner avoiding grudges, resentment, apportioning blame, feelings of revenge, or hate. Try to be more forward looking, with new friends, a new more mature relationship, new happiness, and growth. Think of others rather than your own hurt and anger, especially a new future. Accept divorce as a new beginning, the inevitable pain and change like the pangs of birth. See the ending as painful for both of you, and be grateful for the times you shared and enjoyed together. Be more positive and forward-looking, rather than thinking of the past.

Remedies to consider:-

Ignatia   Indicated for an overwhelming sense of loss and regret leading to depression and loss of confidence.

Natrum mur   A useful remedy for many stress reactions to separation with depression, irritability, and marked fatigue.

Nux vomica   Short-fuse irritability is marked with a zealous determination to impose his own way or to resist inevitable changes. Depressive moods are common.

Kali carb   There are multiple fears and anxieties about the future. Feels irritable, worse for company and often better for being alone.

Sepia   Moods of irritability with depression occur with exhaustion. There is indifference to loved ones.

Staphysagria   There is a tendency to be over-sensitive, resentful, hostile or arrogant, and irritable. Depression with tears of rage is a common feature.

DRUG ABUSE

Drug abuse may occur from prescribed, bought, or illicit drugs, depending upon the individual and his particular type of stress problem. Prescribed drugs are frequently abused to excess, self-prescribed, taken by other members of the family, repeatedly used for the least headache or mild symptom, when originally they were supplied for quite a specific condition. This is particularly common with sedatives and tranquillisers and when used long-term, it is now well known that they may cause severe dependency problems. Abuse can also occur from an excessive or inappropriate use of over-the-counter allergic drugs, especially those which are opiate based and designed for the relief of a chronic cough or acute diarrhoea. The anabolic steroids are known to be widely abused in many sporting events, and during training.

Other bought drugs may also be abused, particularly laxatives, taken to excess for a bowel problem, or misused in an ill-judged attempt to lose weight rapidly.

Stress is the most common underlying cause for abuse of the social drugs, especially alcohol, cigarettes, snuff, coffee and tea.

Heroin, marijuana, cocaine, 'crack', LSD, amphetamine stimulants, tranquillisers, glue or volatile sniffing, also tailor made drugs such as 'ecstasy', are now widely abused by adolescents and adults of all social classes, and have become a major industry. All drugs of abuse are a high risk adventure for every stress sufferer and especially dangerous if mixed as a 'cocktail', taken with alcohol, or in high doses.

Character traits which aggravate the condition

There is lack of confidence, and a tendency for excessive clinging, dependent relationships in many areas of life, but especially close relationships. The same dependency attitudes may also involve food, leading to excesses of coffee, tea, cigarettes and alcohol. At times drug abuse is a way of avoiding closeness and dependency needs. Props are used in many social areas to avoid vulnerability, needing, pain, and problem-solving, at the same time leading to even greater dependency problems.

Practical steps to improve things

Try to take a more overall view, in order to clarify where dependency is a particular problem. Aim to remedy this by being more assertive and creative in these areas, giving rather than taking, or running away. If you are taking several drugs, start by reducing or stopping one of them, preferably one which you know is particularly dangerous or injected. Find someone trusted and neutral to talk to and tell him what you are doing and why. Try to look honestly at the roots of the problem, what has led you into drugs and clarify what you are running from and why. Look more closely at any feelings of rage or anger. If you are not working, try to find some employment, if necessary unpaid voluntary or community work, but try to find something you are interested in, and can contribute to. Make friends with non-drug users, who will not encourage you to continue the habit.

Remedies to consider:-

Lycopodium   This remedy is indicated when there is a tendency to take multiple drugs and supplements because of hypochondriasis.

Nux vomica   Drugs are taken initially to relieve the chronic indigestion and bowel problems, often with excess amounts of coffee, tea, or alcohol.

Opium   There is confusion to the point of delirium with restless agitation. This contrasts with a dream-like state, the mood variable and changeable, easily startled by noise.

Sulphur   A useful remedy to cleanse the system after large amounts of prescribed or bought drugs have been taken.

Thuja   There is irritation with moods of depression. Sensitivity to the least stimulus, living life to extremes, varying from dizzy intoxication to being obstinate, weeping and depression. An important remedy when there are reactions of generalised ill health following long periods of drug abuse.

DUODENAL ULCER

A duodenal ulcer is often a long-standing condition, the outcome of years of bottled-up stress and tension. There is ulceration of the upper duodenal area of the intestine (close to the stomach exit), due to excessive acidity (hydrochloric acid) production, damaging the lining layer cells of this region. It is nearly always associated with chronic stress, and causes pain several hours after eating, typically in the early night hours, and relieved by eating or milk.

The duodenal personality is:- often thin, over-zealous, irritable, excessively competitive, driven by deadlines, irritable (with a short-fuse personality), never able to relax or rest and because of a basic insecurity, unable to stop worrying about work, problems, business and money. The more he tries, the more things seem to go wrong, or he makes mistakes because he tries too hard, is too tense or fatigued, and as a result his judgment is affected. At times he may become desperate and takes a risk or gamble, which usually fails, leading to a loss and even more self-anguish and torture. Pangs of depression occur, and often to an increased intake of alcohol.

Break-up of the marriage is a high risk, because of the pressures. A workaholic, he is never able to relax, or give enough time and attention to the relationship, listen, or come off the telephone. He is a poor sleeper, restless and wakes early, partly because of the high levels of anxiety, and because he drinks too much coffee. He rarely puts on weight, because the stress intensity burns off all surplus energy.

The duodenal personality can be frightening at the car wheel. Impatient, angry with other drivers, he takes risks, cutting in to save a few seconds, without having any real reason to do so or knowing how to use the time gained at so much peril. He complains a great deal about life, never feels really fit or well, yet rarely rests or takes a holiday except under pressure. Because of the intensity of competitive feelings, problems of suspicion or jealousy tend to occur, and he is never an easy relaxed person to be with.

Character traits which aggravate the condition
There is a tendency to worry excessively and not to let go of problems, at the same time, too private and not open enough with others, failing to share feelings, needs, and thoughts. Usually distant and a loner, a major source of the duodenal irritability is being over-competitive and constantly driven by deadlines. Depression with irritability and never relaxing, leads eventually to 'burn-out' or total exhaustion.

Practical steps to improve things
Aim to be more open with others. Share more and let go of feelings and thoughts. Try to be more trusting with a more open expression of you as a person. Start with a few people, perhaps giving out in certain selected areas and then broaden these. Be more open with your partner. Don't keep feelings in, or delay talking about your problems or emotions. Exercise regularly, eating little and often, but especially eating slowly. Try to be more relaxed when eating, and avoid getting irritable at the table. If you have developed rigid controls, tight schedules and self-imposed deadlines, try to modify and soften these attitudes. Practise regular periods of relaxation, yoga, or meditation.

Remedies to consider:-

Arsenicum   The temperament is fastidious, neat and over-controlled. All symptoms are worse in the early night hours after midnight.

Carbo veg   There are major problems of flatulence and pain, mainly in the upper abdominal area, aggravated by heat. Feels constantly full of wind and exhausted, with no drive or energy. All symptoms are worse for eating fatty food, coffee, or alcohol.

Lycopodium   There is upper abdominal discomfort with gassy indigestion. All symptoms are worse in the late afternoon or early evening.

Natrum mur   There is considerable stress anxiety with tension, heartburn, and sweating when eating. Thirst is always marked and salty foods are craved. Worse from heat.

Nux vomica   Irritability with tension leads to chronic problems of indigestion and constipation. Nausea and flatulence, with a bitter taste.

Ornithogalum A very useful remedy for chronic duodenal problems with nausea, distention, and fatigue.

79

DYSMENORRHOEA

Painful period colic may be partly caused by hormonal imbalance, but it is often related to underlying emotional problems. Stress is not usually the direct result of the period discomfort, but often precedes it. Any irritability or tension is made worse because feelings are more on the surface at the time of menstruation.

Problems may occur in women of any age who are menstruating, but it is particularly common after a relationship break-up or crisis. The periods are often irregular, heavy, or dribbling, and may contain clots for a day or two until the full flow finally starts, usually bringing relief from pain and discomfort. Spasms of colicky pain are mainly due to contraction of the uterine muscles combined with circulatory stasis in the pelvic area. There may be a period of pre-menstrual tension (PMT), feeling tired, moody, irritable, before the start of the cycle, and sometimes unwell for two weeks out of every four.

Low backache is a common complaint, the result of pelvic congestion and stasis (very slow movement of the circulation) in the uterine veins, causing heaviness and depression. There is often a drop in levels of libidinal interest as a result of feeling tired, bloated, and unattractive.

Shedding tears usually brings some relief from the underlying tension and tends to occur anyway, but is particularly common whenever understanding or sympathy are shown. The reason why closeness is rebuffed at this time, is often a feeling that if she starts to cry, she will not be able to control her emotions and cry for the whole week. There is a mistaken sense of needing to maintain all the controls which can lead to alienation within the couple. The husband or partner may not really fully understand what is wrong and why the woman feels irritable, her increased need for attention, to be held, for company, help, support, and especially affection at this time. If there is a failure of meaningful discussion between the couple, this adds to any frustration or depression, leading to alienation, heightening tension and anxiety, aggravating the menstrual problem which sometimes feels like an incurable mess. If the underlying stress problems are relieved, the woman can relax more which helps the pelvic circulation to be re-established.

Character traits which aggravate the condition
A tendency to be tense, or to worry excessively and not relaxing sufficiently, quickly feeling under pressure, and then becoming irritable. Fear and anxiety further aggravate the problems.

Practical steps to improve things
Exercise regularly to stimulate the pelvic circulation and to encourage bowel elimination, especially before and during your period. You may benefit from quite vigorous exercise, e.g. walking quickly or swimming. If you are overweight, adjust your weight to target levels for your age and height. Try to relax as much as possible, especially just before and during period times, aiming to be as open and spontaneous as you can at other times of the month. Especially avoid holding problems in by denying or suppressing feelings and emotions.

Remedies to consider:-

Belladonna There are heavy, painful periods, coming on too soon. The pains are sharp, sudden, and darting, causing a flush of heat with sweating. Restless agitation is a feature.

Lilium tig There is an anxious agitated state with depression, worse for consolation. Irritability is marked. The uterus feels heavy, with a dragging-down discomfort.

Magnesium phos One of the best remedies for menstrual colic.

Nux vomica The pains are spasmodic, especially in the low back sacral region. Irritability is marked.

Pulsatilla For mainly left-sided uterine pain. The periods are heavy or delayed, with variable drawing or pressure pains in the uterus.

Sepia The main symptoms are a dragging-down, heavy pelvic discomfort, with low back pain, irritability, fatigue, and indifference to loved ones.

ECZEMA

Depending on its severity and the area of the body affected, eczema can be a very distressing stress-related skin condition which may occur at any age. It is characterised by dry itchy patches, often red or raised, with irregular irritated areas which have a tendency to weep, crack, or become infected. Bleeding may occur, especially if the eczema is scratched.

In most cases the exact causes are not clear. There is often believed to be an allergic cause, but if skin tests are carried out, there is usually a very wide range of sensitivities, including:- house dust mite, animal-hair, moulds, pollens and foodstuffs. There is rarely one specific substance which is triggering off the eczema, and desensitization does not always lead to a cure.

A common factor in the majority of eczema sufferers is that they are too tense or oversensitive and often contain an enormous amount of repressed anger and irritability, which is intensified by the skin condition. Aggressive, often damaging scratching tends to cause a secondary infection and perpetuates the condition. The typical eczema sufferer is usually a person with ability and potential, but because he is over-anxious, he tends to anticipate problems. He often works in spurts rather than in a consistent way, not achieving his full potential because of lack of confidence, not trying hard enough because he expects to fail, or not to cope in some way.

Eczema is nearly always temporarily improved by a holiday or a change of environment. It is aggravated by any stress or pressure situation. An examination, change of school or job, an impending interview, fear of redundancy, all tend to worsen the eczema, causing it to become more angry and intensely irritating. It is often better for warm mild weather, sunlight, sea air and sea bathing. In the writer's experience, the long-term use of steroids is not helpful, sometimes leading to chronic eczema problems, the rash held just under the skin and irritable, neither disappearing or progressing in any positive way. Because any underlying psychological problems are not touched by steroids, the eczema tends to extend into new areas, spreading up the body.

Character traits which aggravate the condition

There is an excessive nervousness and tension, with over-sensitivity to others. Shyness, withdrawal, fear of disapproval, are common and there is a tendency to hold back with feelings. Alienation or unpopularity, is often due to the lack of confidence, keeping others at a distance. High levels of anxiety may build up, especially about being approved of and accepted, creating fear and tension.

Practical steps to improve things

Eat a sensible bland wholesome diet, avoiding spicy, rich, sweet foods. Especially avoid sweets, chocolate bars, ice cream, sweet biscuits or cakes. Aim to reduce weight, and if this has increased recently, bring it down to target levels for your height and age. Avoid allowing anxiety levels to build-up, by talking to your family, friends, or partner more openly about any issues or fears which concern you. If you can't talk with your partner or family, talk to a friend, but don't withdraw from others, or become excessively preoccupied with your skin problems, or what might happen. Aim to be more open and spontaneous. Avoid scratching, or picking at any eczema areas to prevent infection.

Remedies to consider:-

Arsenicum   The skin is dry, cracked, and scaly, the irritation worse in the early night hours, at 1-3.00 am.

Belladonna   The skin feels burning hot, red, dry, and is often infected, causing a high temperature. Restless agitation is a feature.

Formica   There is a violent 'tickling' irritation of the area affected. Most symptoms are worse on the left side of the body.

Graphites   The skin is dry and cracked, oozing a clear yellow discharge. There may be moods of tearful irritability.

Psorinum   The eczema is irritated and dirty-looking with a crusty eczema. Lack of energy and always feeling chilly.

Rhus tox   The skin is irritated, red, swollen and often infected, better for heat and fresh air.

Sulphur   There is a burning, irritating chronic eczema problem, with an offensive discharge of pus or clear fluid, worse for contact with water.

85

EXAMINATION FEARS

These are common fears at any age. When they have already occurred in adolescence or childhood, they may re-appear in the adult during the course of a particular stress situation - before a job interview, a change of job, or a group in-training day.

The parents themselves may have lacked confidence, although never openly admitted it, but fearing a competitive situation because they anticipated a challenge or a humiliation. A child can often sense these fears within the parents and react to them, in this way sowing the seeds of future anxiety. A common fear is of 'freezing', or losing all memory functioning in an examination situation. Also feeling faint or weak, having an attack of diarrhoea, feeling sick, or becoming panicky under pressure and having to walk out.

Often the exact causes are not clear. A child is nervous from a young age, or lacks experience with others of his age. He may have had an overprotected upbringing, or made to feel awkward in some way which undermines confidence. In many cases, he has never learned how best to tackle an examination situation, to lay-out and plan, or how much time to give to each question. There is often a lack of strategy which undermines confidence and experience. Above all there is an exaggeration and a distortion of the whole examination situation, creating intolerable pressures which create blocks to memory and a relaxed response.

The problem of 'examination nerves' may have originated months or years ago, anticipating unreasonable high standards which are impossible to meet, at the same time undermining confidence and fluency. If there is a strong sense of guilt or inadequacy, this can lead to a reluctance to confide the problem to the family, other students or the tutor.

'Examination nerves' responds well to homoeopathy, helping to reduce anxiety levels and strengthening the natural drives and abilities of the individual. Often, fear of failure is given too much prominence, making every test situation a nightmare. Every aspect of life, including an examination situation, needs to be kept in perspective, if not, it becomes distorted and self-destructive, allowing panic to occur and fears which may totally undermine performance. If there is severe anticipatory anxiety with distortion, homoeopathy can help bring this back into reality and perspective.

Character traits which aggravate the condition

There is a tendency to exaggerate, not keeping things in perspective, with fear of failure or disapproval. Life is seen in bits, or in isolation, rather than as an overall meaningful totality. There is a tendency to exaggerate the importance of isolated incidents and to be far too anxious and fearful.

Practical steps to improve things

Try to think more broadly and creatively in your approach to problems. See life as a chain of events, and not just as isolated ones. Practise your exam technique well in advance, so that you can confidently use the allotted time to your advantage. Be well prepared, but not excessively so. Don't see failure or a 're-sit' as a disaster. It could be to your advantage. Work steadily throughout the year. Revise early, after each term and relax more. Meditation may also help.

87

Remedies to consider:-

Aconitum   There is an acute fear reaction, with restless agitation.

Argentum nit Phobic anxiety is marked, with impulsive tendencies, worse from any form of heat.

Gelsemium   For mild 'examination nerves'. He is lethargic and prefers to be alone.

Lycopodium   Anticipatory anxiety is marked, with restlessness and fear. Self-confidence is low.

Natrum mur   There is a problem of tearful depression and low motivation, lacking confidence in all social situations and never relaxed or at ease with others.

Pulsatilla   There are many very varied anxiety symptoms, but always feeling worse from heat. Tearful and hypochondriacal, he is very fearful of all tests, feeling tense and trapped in any kind of pressure situation.

FAINTING AND WEAKNESS

This is a common symptom, often reflecting nervous exhaustion, tension and anguish, or sometimes due to a fear reaction, draining energy reserves because of a sustained adrenalin release, and aggravated by exhaustion and failure to relax or sleep.

Fear and tension, the conviction of some impending disaster, may cause frightening dreams or nightmares which drain energy because they undermine rest during sleep. If stress levels are high, food levels may not sufficiently sustain the body, and often there is constant hunger which neither increases body weight or energy levels. Loss of weight may occur from nervous strain, aggravated by smoking, or endless cups of coffee or tea, and often undermining the vital energy of the stomach and the lungs, depressing the nervous system. There may be a terrifying sense of impending doom, collapse or disaster, even of imminent death.

Sometimes fainting is more a symptom of a hysterical condition. The person, indeed the whole life situation, is highly dramatic. He may be deathly pale, sweating, with a marble almost greenish hue to the face, seemingly at death's door, yet somehow surviving and remaining alert and aware. Moods and emotions seem to shift and change, at the same time as directing others even from the floor, gathering attention and court around him and finally rallying with a complete inexplicable recovery without explanation and having refused all attempts at medical help. The fainting attacks are often familiar to the close family, who may have seen several similar situations over the years, and always following the same dramatic course.

Hysterical faints tend to occur at the most inconvenient moment when everyone is busy; in a hurry to complete a deadline; perhaps catch a plane or train; often just before a major change in the family dynamics; the annual holiday; before a change of job or house, a theatre outing, dinner party, school meeting, or any event which is important and where there is a high level of pressure, tension and anxiety. The faint takes all the attention until it there is recovery by an apparently miracle cure, and usually no-one dares to move or leave until this has happened.

Character traits which aggravate the condition
There is a tendency to panic, to see things in extremes, to suppress needs, wishes and feelings, so that they build-up into unreal expectations and then expanding into excessive tension. All of this causes weakness, often fainting or inertia.

Practical steps to improve things
Don't anticipate disasters quite so much, live more in the present and in reality, rather than feeling that your whole existence is on a knife-edge. If you are constantly expecting a disaster in every aspect of life, you will always be trying to survive, to avoid 'going over the edge', and always tense. If you feel faint, try to sit down before it happens. Avoid stuffy atmospheres, but don't anticipate fainting and try to relax more in all social crowd situations. Practise meditation, yoga or relaxation during the day. Consider a relaxation tape if you need any extra help to let go of tension.

Remedies to consider:-

China   Profuse sweating occurs with a variable temperature. There is weakness, fainting, with exhaustion of the whole body, worse for movement.

Gelsemium   Fear, dullness, and apathy are marked features which drain energy and lead to exhaustion.

Nux moschata   There is a drowsy weakness, especially of the knees and exhaustion after dressing. Complains of feeling faint and nauseated.

Phosphoric ac   Weakness, apathy and prostration are worse in the morning, There is a strong desire to stay in bed in order to rest, and because of lack of strength.

Phosphorus   Extreme sensitivity, lack of confidence, depression and fear, create a tendency to faint. This is due to excess emotion.

Pulsatilla   All the emotions are excessive and variable, from tears to laughter, anger or fainting. Always feels worse for heat and there is an absence of thirst.

FATIGUE

This is one of the most common symptoms of any stress condition, and sometimes may be the only symptom. But however stress manifests, with the exception of an overactive state of nerves (when energy is boundless), fatigue, tiredness, a jaded unwell feeling is almost always present. The symptom tends to persist throughout the day, and typically fatigue is present on waking, after rest, and sometimes on holiday. It is often accompanied by anxiety, often felt as 'butterflies in the stomach', and despite going to bed early and sleeping late, there may still be a sense of not feeling rested, and only fallen asleep five minutes before the alarm went off.

Exhaustion is usually present throughout the day and does not vary much, except that it is worse before going out, seeing friends or family, the noise and demands of the children, or from any demand for help and attention, or when there is a change in routine.

Where a particular area of the body is affected, for example the chest (weakness, shortage of breath, sighing breathing or tightness), the heart (with palpitations, chest fullness, often a rapid pulse), energy levels tend to drop at different times, for example the lung and chest, in the early night hours, 1-3.00 am. Heat tends to aggravate the fatigue, and it is often worse in the late afternoon or evening, or when a meal is delayed or missed.

Fatigue may make you over-tired, and exhausted, longing to sleep, yet consistently restless, either too hot or too cold and never comfortable or at ease.

Character traits which aggravate the condition

There is a tendency to be continually anxious, tense, and controlled or under pressure. All of this holds down the free expression of emotion and depletes energy and drive, leading to exhaustion, irritability, and an overwhelming sense of frustration.

Practical steps to improve things

Aim to talk much more about your personal feelings as soon as you experience them, but don't let them take over the whole of you as exaggerated fears or fantasies. Avoid letting feelings build-up to an extreme degree so that you cannot relax or switch off. The energy required to keep the 'lid' on feelings will drain all your reserves. Practise letting go from time to time and deep relaxation some time during the day. Overall, aim to be more **you**, for more of the time, and don't avoid or be afraid to say what you think and feel. Also try not to spare the feelings of others at the expense of your personal self-expression. If later you feel that you have gone too far, then you can always apologise.

Remedies to consider:-

Arnica   There is a sense of feeling bruised psychologically, creating exhaustion and fatigue.

Cuprum met   Loss of weight occurs with restless trembling and agitation. There is a marked sense of unease, the limbs feeling weak.

Ferrum phos   For fatigue and lack of energy, often shortness of breath. There is a nervous, sensitive temperament, the face flushed.

Graphites   For weakness and exhaustion of the whole body. Nausea is present, the abdomen distended. Also for dull stomach pains.

Kali phos   A useful remedy for weakness and exhaustion.

Nux moschata   There is a chilly drowsiness, the mouth dry. Fainting turns are a frequent occurrence.

Opium   For drowsiness with exhaustion, and severe constipation.

Phosphoric ac   Weakness and prostration are marked, worse in the morning. Lacks ideas or drive. There is a dry and ticklish evening cough.

FEAR

To some extent, fear is present in every stress condition. It often first manifests as a loss of confidence, reluctance to go out, feeling nervous about meeting others, fear of new situations or anything unfamiliar or new. There is a tendency to be inhibited, to hold back because of lack of confidence, being seen as nervous or tense, and often a fear of fear itself or what it might do. The sense of fear may be worse in any new social situation where you feel vulnerable, unfamiliar and unsure of yourself. There may also be fear of any new form of self-expression - changing clothes, or hair style, going out shopping, making contact with others. A man may fear meeting or talking to women, partly fearing any underlying excitement or sexual interest, as well as an impulse to run away. Fear and envy of other men may occur because he feels they are more interesting, talk more, are younger, more sexually appealing, intelligent, have a more rewarding job, a good-looking partner, more money, a nicer car or home. A strong competitive instinct causes many of the problems, because of the way success is seen, and often how poorly he rates his own achievements.

There may also be an underlying sense of inadequacy, which is never really admitted or discussed. This may be based on lack of social experience or assertiveness, the ability to be fluent in speech and ideas. Fear is often fed by this kind of very self-destructive imagery, based on the past, a tendency to be over critical and damaging self-confidence. A chance insensitive remark may have been made at school, but leaving a scar on confidence.

Stress fear is often linked to an over-evaluation of others. Far too much emphasis is put on superficial impressions, comparison, sometimes at the most trivial level. Often the individual is extremely able or gifted, but lacks the confidence, drive and ability to go out and use his talents, to follow them through into a tangible reality.

Character traits which aggravate the condition
There is a tendency to control and withhold any feelings of rage and aggression. This then feeds any unconscious aggressive destructive fantasies, almost confirming them and adding to fears, because anger has not been tested (expressed) in a reality situations.

Practical steps to improve things
Try not to allow feelings of anger, rage, frustration, irritability and resentment to accumulate. Let the feelings come out and be expressed as they occur. Most fear is directed at external situations, i.e. fear of crowds, heights, open spaces, people, closeness, being hurt, fear of death, or madness. It may also attach itself, to quite ordinary everyday happenings and turn them into a threat, e.g. fear of supermarkets, eating, washing, touching certain objects. Try to give yourself more time to slowly assess the logic of a particular fear situation. The symptoms are nearly always symbolic of inner tensions and anxieties, resembling the anxiety which occurs in dreams. Aim to reduce feelings of being trapped or limited, by keeping yourself stretched and stimulated psychologically, with new interests, drives, friends, and contacts.

Remedies to consider:-

Aconitum A remedy for restlessness and agitation, associated with fearful apprehensive moods, especially of death or the future.

Arsenicum Feeling exhausted, always cold, restless, anxious to the point of despair. Obsessional fears, and remote from all close social contacts.

Kali carb Depression with anxiety and fatigue. All symptoms are worse in the early hours, from 3-5.00.

Lycopodium A remedy for fear of the future, causing stress anxiety or depressive problems and severe lack of confidence.

Natrum mur Thin, covered with sweat, craving salt, he is severely depressed and tearful, worse for any close contact with others or consolation.

Phosphorus Over-sensitivity accounts for much of the restless anxiety and fears. He is constantly looking for acceptance and reassurance.

FRIGIDITY

Frigidity is vaginal spasm during intercourse and due to the association of apprehension, anxiety, and tension with the sexual act. It is a common problem in immature girls, with lack of social contact or experience with males, and particularly where sexuality has become the object of too much fantasy without involvement with a male partner to bring it into balance and reality. It may sometimes occur when overtired, or nervous, with insufficient time to relax, feel at ease and comfortable, where intercourse has been imposed (or only accepted because of fear), without a close affectionate trusting relationship. If the physical side of a relationship becomes over-emphasised and given more importance than the emotional side, this can lead to a sense of not being fully involved. Feelings of unreality or alienation may cause problems, often because the more affectionate aspects of the relationship are not expressed.

Where problems are discussed in a caring, sensitive way, as part of the couple's relationship, this inevitably leads to greater trust and relaxation. If frigidity persists, it usually helps to talk about it, without creating a pressure situation, trying to understand what makes it better or worse. It is helpful to look at any stress problem in this way, because it strengthens trust, gives a greater sense of involvement, understanding and sharing, a feeling that the partner really does care.

When problems are not talked about openly, then guilt or shame may be reinforced, leading to a build-up of anxiety. Problems are likely to become worse because of increasing fear, tension and fear of failure.

If the frigidity remains persistent and difficult, not significantly improved by sensitive, open discussion combined with homoeopathy, focal counselling, or help from a specialised sexual therapist may be required.

It is always important to prevent intimacy and sexuality from becoming demanding or pressurised. Like all aspects of life, the sexual act must be allowed to be spontaneous, find its own natural rhythm. It should not be controlled, but allowed to develop at its own pace and in its own time.

Character traits which aggravate the condition
Anticipation of failure or pain causes tension and spasm. There is a tendency to withhold, to defend against a possible hurt, rejection or humiliation, by holding-in tightly in all areas. Fantasy life may dominate the reality assessment of your partner, especially a new relationship where you feel vulnerable. There is often an excessive fear of others, apprehension of close contact, and lack of confidence.

Practical steps to improve things
Try to perceive the sexual act as a simple and natural act of union, which you are distorting by imposing tension and anxiety. Be much more relaxed overall, not anticipating problems or difficulties. Practise gentle quiet relaxation, stroking and holding your partner, instead of full intercourse, to take the pressure off. Aim to broaden the problem away from a specific sexual difficulty and try to see how you are tensing up in other situations. This will help you relax and reduce tension. Try to avoid sexualizing broader tension problems, as this may worsen them. Practice regular relaxation and consider meditation as a further step to reduce anxiety.

Remedies to consider:-

Agnus cast   The mood is one of sadness and remoteness, absent minded. The sexual act is felt to be repulsive.

Natrum mur   A useful remedy for frigidity problems when associated with depression or severe anxiety. The skin is cold, and covered in sweat, all symptoms worse for sea air. Salt is craved.

Phosphorus   Frigidity is caused by being tense, anxious, failure to relax and over-sensitivity. Always feeling cold, yet craves ice cold drinks.

Pulsatilla   For variable frigidity problems, with tears and changeable moods, worse for heat. Thirst is absent.

Sepia   Fatigue, low backache, heavy periods with clots and dragging down pains, indifference to loved ones and depression, are some of the major symptom indications for this remedy.

Silicea   The main problem is lack of confidence and fear of failure. There is a tendency to sweat profusely, always chilly and better for heat.

FROZEN SHOULDER

This is a painful often stress-related condition, usually triggered by a stiff or sudden movement when in a state of pressure, tension or anxiety. An often insignificant action, perhaps lifting a cup from the table, or reaching down to floor level, causes either acute pain and discomfort, or an intermittent ache with limitation of shoulder movement, especially reaching to the back area. There is spasm of the surrounding ligaments protecting the shoulder from a mild tendon inflammatory reaction. Often the onset is far from clear, and the condition comes on slowly over the course of a few days, but usually at a time of stress, when doing too much or where there is a crisis in the family or at work. Some of the typical problems which lead to a frozen shoulder are the break-up of a marriage, the threat of redundancy or early retirement, anxiety about illness of a close member of the family where the outcome is uncertain. At such times there is a greater tendency to become accident-prone, because of underlying frustration and feelings of guilt.

The condition may lead to constant discomfort and stiffness, frequently worse at night, interrupting sleep and often better for lying on the affected shoulder and improved by heat. A frozen shoulder always causes some degree of movement limitation, with difficulty lifting the arm high, to reach up behind the head (to brush the hair), also behind the upper back (to fasten a bra strap). It does not usually affect both shoulders. If not treated, the condition may last for weeks or months and undermine health, leading to feelings of depression.

The underlying emotional pressure is clearly seen by an increased tendency to short-fuse irritability, mood-swings, restless shallow sleep, sometimes early waking. Part of the problem may be a compulsive need to do everything in a hurry, as if being chased (usually quite unconsciously, by a strict over-demanding conscience, and linked to upbringing and parental attitudes). Because too many things are being done at once, there is insufficient time to be paced and rhythmic, leading to poorly co-ordinated or ill-judged movements and tension, which causes damage.

Character traits which aggravate the condition
There is a tendency to be rigid and stiff in all attitudes, holding-in feelings and spontaneity, without ever letting go and often because of fear and a need to control self and others.

Practical steps to improve things
Practise being easy and much more relaxed throughout the day, letting go of all body tension, and not just in the shoulder area. Aim to release emotions and feelings more openly and spontaneously. Avoid locking yourself up tightly behind a facade of invulnerability and conforming 'niceness'. If you feel irritable, anxious, unhappy, or concerned, then say so to your partner or family. Start now, by freeing your mind and your emotions. In this way, your shoulder will also improve and your accident-proneness in the future. But make this a way of life, not just a technique you are trying for a week or so.

Remedies to consider:-

Arnica
There is a bruised, swollen, painful shoulder, aggravated by movement, cold or damp air.

Calcarea sulph
The shoulder is stiff on waking with discomfort in the area. There is a sharp darting pain when putting a coat on.

Ledum
The shoulder is heavy, with a tearing pain on movement, the area bruised and sore. Symptoms are worse on the right side, and in the morning.

Natrum sulph
A remedy for left-sided problems, sensitive to changes of weather and barometric pressure. Better for warm, dry air, worse for cold or damp.

Rhus tox
The shoulder is stiff and painful, all symptoms worse on waking, and better in the evening, from heat and movement.

Ruta
The shoulder feels bruised and painful, worse at night when lying down, from cold or damp.

Sanguinaria
A useful remedy for right-sided problems, worse for touch and movement.

103

HEADACHE

This is one of the commonest of all stress symptoms and may occur in any part of the head, but it is particularly associated with tension across the forehead, temple area and upper-neck region. Where tension is the underlying problem, there may be clenching of the jaw, or teeth-grinding, often occurring in sleep. The headaches are often very variable, tending to move around, worse after a weekend or a holiday break, or first thing in the morning. They are also worse:- from chatter and noise, bright lights, contact with people, when feeling rushed or tired, after eating, before a period, after alcohol, from driving, and especially when tired.

Stress headaches are worse from any form of environmental irritation, including traffic fumes, the office environment, central heating, dry recycled air, stale cigarette smoke, cooking or perfume smells, or where the office does not receive natural daylight and fresh air from an open window.

The modern open-plan office with many people and constant noise and movement, can lead to claustrophobic feelings, trapped or swamped by the coming and going, lack of daylight, or a free circulation of air.

Temporary relief may be gained by drinking strong coffee or tea, smoking, or alcohol. But these usually give minimal help, and may undermine health, causing nausea, heartburn, palpitations, a dry mouth, sweating, feeling faint, or a lack of appetite.

A stress headache may be the result of a dispute, or tense emotional situation, either at home or work. Although usually better for a rest or a weekend break, they may be worse if overtired, and are sometimes aggravated by the relaxation or family demands. As the stress pressures are taken off, there may be an increase of irritability, impatience, tension, and head or neck discomfort. This is because of the time it takes to relax and because a longer time is needed to wind down and relax fully.

Stress headaches tend to recur over a period of months or years, causing a loss of enjoyment of life, often short-fuse irritability and depression. The tensions undermine social relationships, concentration, work output, libido, and a more enjoyable creative life-style.

Migraine headaches usually settle over one eye, and are associated with vomiting, and light sensitivity.

Character traits which aggravate the condition
There is usually a combination of excessive tension, anger, and uneasy self-control, especially in stress situations or where a new or unfamiliar event is anticipated. Irritability is often a feature, but like all the emotions, it is held tightly inside.

Practical steps to improve things
Aim to be more at ease with yourself as well as with others. A fifteen minute period of twice daily relaxation is helpful. Always clarify any 'trigger' areas of stress or emotion which bring on the headaches, and try to understand why these particularly upset you. Aim to be more open and spontaneous with ideas, and the expression of feelings.

Remedies to consider:-

Aconitum For violent acute headaches, with restlessness, fear, and agitation.

Glonoine There is a throbbing headache, with dizziness, worse for covering the head.

Kali carb A cutting left-sided headache occurs, worse from cold air. Anxiety, depression and fatigue.

Lachesis For left-sided headache, worse on waking and after sleep. Over-talkative, worse for tight clothing.

Lycopodium Indicated for right-sided head pain, worse from 4-8.00 pm, and often related to anticipatory fears.

Natrum mur The headaches are stress-related, associated with severe moods of tearful depression and anxiety.

Nux vomica There are spasms of pain with dizziness, worse on waking, for noise or bright light.

Pulsatilla The headache is variable, with mood variations, worse for heat.

Silicea The pain is at the back of the head with dizziness, improved if the head is kept covered.

IMPOTENCE

Weakness or failure of the male erection is a common symptom of fatigue, anxiety or pressure, and occurs in most men at some time. The problem often happens because of not being at ease or comfortable in a particular relationship, feelings of guilt, or that you are expected to perform, when in reality you would rather relax, talk, do nothing, or sleep for a few hours. Masculine potency is very sensitive to any form of stress or pressure.

Occasional loss of erection is normal, and really it is unimportant. Far too much social importance and pressure is put on the male for a reliable and sustained erection in all circumstances, especially when there is a new partner. Ideal role models, such as the James Bond image of instant sustainable libido, exerts pressure on the masculine ego, undermining confidence. What matters is not trying to be another 007 but to be yourself, relaxed, authentic, and not acting or pretending, genuinely interested and caring for the other person. Having to live up to an unattainable role model, means a weakening of personal integrity and self-confidence, and with this comes sexual anxiety and male potency problems.

Impotence is more rarely associated with an actual physical condition, such as diabetes, or degenerative nervous conditions, for example multiple sclerosis. It may however occur as a side-effect of a prescribed drug (especially the beta-blockers), or follow using anti-depressants, and some tranquillisers.

A man became inhibited, when his grown-up children were in the house at the time of having intercourse, in case they could hear what was happening. Sensitivity about noise is a common problem and often points to oversensitivity in other areas. There may be fear or anxiety at making any kind of noise, being overheard, laughed at, feeling foolish, especially if less inhibited or excessive in some way. This is usually because of a confidence problem, and putting too much weight on what others may think.

Many men feel a failure if they do not achieve a mutual orgasm each time, holding back, when the woman is not fully aroused, yet not discussing with her how she feels at the time, or explicit about their arousal fantasies, erotic areas, and what gives pleasure. Men are more likely to achieve an orgasm during each act of intercourse than a woman, who also experiences pleasure by identifying with the male orgasm and his enjoyment of the sexual act. At times the woman is more ready, and both do reach an orgasm together. But this is bound to vary with each new and different act of intercourse, the quality of the union, and the sharing, and where she is in her cycle. The male should never think of himself as a machine, and the variables depend on the couple, how well they play, share, and communicate together, also upon their level of physical fitness.

The male may wake with an erection, feel aroused and want to have intercourse. His partner may be less aroused in the mornings (but more so in the evening), but she would nevertheless enjoy the experience of him inside the vagina. If the male obsessionally tries to arouse the female and does not know that it is the wrong time of the day or month, or she is still tired or half-asleep, he can easily create a destructive pattern, and lose confidence. He may then start to believe he is failing in some way. The truth may be that he is looking for failure, or proof of it, because this has been a familiar pattern throughout his life, which he either expects or fears.

Looking for confirmation of either success or failure is essentially selfish and narcissistic, and may be the underlying reason for a potency problems to occur. Once the male is more mature, able to talk and discuss, share both affection and fears, then the variations in male erection can be accepted as a normal part of a global psychological whole, just one aspect of overall togetherness and intimacy.

Character traits which aggravate the condition
There is a tendency to worry too much over trifles, to be over-concerned about details, appearance and performance generally. Beneath the excessive concern is often a childhood fear of disapproval or rejection.

Practical steps to improve things
Try to reduce tension throughout the day, and don't rush into situations. Aim to see how you do this in various situations, leading to exhaustion or impaired performance in other areas, than the narrow sexual one. Regular relaxation sessions are helpful, also meditation or yoga. Try also to be less concerned about how others judge you with more emphasis on being natural, really just being you. Stop smoking, if you are using this to relieve tension during the day, as it will aggravate the problem. At the same time avoid any weight increase. Discuss any worries openly with your partner.

Remedies to consider:-

Agnus cast   There is weakness, with an absence of sexual desire, associated with depression, lack of self-confidence, and exhaustion.

Argentum nit   The thought of intercourse causes anxiety. Worse from heat.

Arnica   The impotence is transitory, and associated with feeling hurt or bruised.

Lycopodium   Lack of self-confidence causes every aspect of life to be rushed and precipitate. This may lead to premature ejaculation. Great fear of failure, and of the future.

Natrum mur   Anxiety, and a tearful depression with weakness, causes a very low libidinal drive.

Pulsatilla   There is a variable libidinal drive because of underlying fear, lack of confidence and extremes of emotion.

Silicea   Useful when the whole body is covered with sweat, and often exhausted, cold and thin. Fear of failure undermines both drive and confidence.

INDIGESTION

This is a common stress manifestation, often caused by excessive pressure, with high levels of anxiety and repressed emotional feelings, especially rage and anger. The underlying intensity of emotions is given little or no direct outlet, causing an outpouring of excess hydrochloric acid into the stomach, which results in pain, wind, heartburn, nausea, irritability and often a bloated, heavy, leaden feeling, which is sometimes described as a 'hot bubble' sensation in the upper stomach.

When living in a situation of constant tension, it is common for the stomach to be adversely affected in some way. Almost any form of stress (but especially rage, fear or tension), affects the lining wall of the stomach, causing the blood vessels to dilate and affects normal gastric functioning.

If high levels of acid are constantly released into the stomach, a breakdown of the lining mucosa may be inevitable, leading to peptic ulceration. Sometimes the erosion perforates a blood vessel causing severe bleeding. If the contents of the stomach enter the abdominal cavity, peritonitis may occur with very severe pain, shock and collapse.

Most stress tension is felt in the stomach or solar plexus, with a sinking feeling of discomfort, and a heavy dragging-down sensation. If gastric functioning continues to be undermined, it may affect the entire digestive process, leading to loss of weight, diarrhoea, nausea, vomiting, and often anaemia.

Pain from gastric irritation may be felt at the tip of one or other shoulder, also in the upper back region and along the spinal column. Discomfort may also be experienced in the lower abdomen, usually on the left side along the colon, or large bowel region, especially when constipation is a problem. There is often a foul taste in the mouth, the tongue coated with a thick, yellow or brown covering, offensive breath and constant hunger. Loud burps, offensive wind and indigestion are frequent, worse when hungry, and also after eating.

Character traits which aggravate the condition
The major problem is a tendency to hold feelings down far too tightly, with all stress tensions referred to the body. Particularly the alimentary (digestive) tract is involved forming excessive amounts of acid, which slow down the digestive process and encourage fermentation and eventually ulceration.

Practical steps to improve things
Aim to be more relaxed when eating, not rushing or bolting your food, tasting, enjoying and relishing what you are eating to encourage the digestive process to be more healthy and less painful. You may have a great deal of internal turmoil, perhaps a tendency to be short-fuse and impatient, too easily irritated. Try talking much earlier about feelings, before they build up to form a rock-hard solid lump in the stomach area, and exercise regularly. Eat less, but eat more slowly, taking double the amount of time and chewing twice as much as usual. If there is still an area of tension, try to resolve this by looking at the realities, and not allowing yourself to be carried away by fantasies of disasters, or what might happen. Avoid all alcohol until the problem has improved, and then drink in moderation.

Remedies to consider:-

Calcarea   There is a sour tasting indigestion, with sweating, nausea, lack of energy, and feeling cold. Usually overweight and anxious, often obsessional in behaviour. Always feeling better for heat.

Carbo veg   Flatulence and upper abdominal distention is marked. Better for cold air, and intolerant of heat.

Ipecacuanha   Overweight and weak, there is irritability, with constant nausea and often vomiting.

Lycopodium   There is a windy flatulence with distention of the upper stomach area. All symptoms are worse in the afternoon and early evening, or if a meal is missed.

Nux vomica   Irritability is marked with spasms of pain, also nausea and vomiting. There are chronic constipation problems. There is a craving for rich fatty foods.

Ornithogalum For chronic indigestion problems, with wind and pain. Depressive mood swings, often completely exhausted.

113

RECURRENT INFECTIONS

These often have a link with acute or chronic stress conditions, which deplete the vital energy reserves and immune resistance levels of the body, so that infections of fungal, viral, or bacterial origin, are more likely to occur. They are particularly common in those who work with the public and have high stress levels. Teachers, nurses, taxi drivers, are especially vulnerable, or those working in noisy confined places, often excessively warm, and where the air quality is poor.

Pollution and allergy are major factors which play an important role in undermining vital resistance and vitality; especially dust, sulphur dioxide and nitrogen dioxide, which undermine chest health, mainly due to exhaust emissions from cars and lorries in our cities.

But whatever the physical exposure, stress is nearly always a relevant factor in repeated infections. High levels of emotion, undermine and drain overall resistance, and make you more prone to infection. Stress, tension, pressures from the environment, or any form of sustained anxiety, makes you more susceptible to infection. This is basically because the subtle defensive energies which surround the body are weakened, allowing penetration of weak or vulnerable areas, especially following a recent illness, accident, or operation. An example might be where the tonsils have been removed in the past, leading to a higher incidence of recurrent throat infections. Also following glandular fever, or where there is a long-standing spinal misalignment.

Homoeopathy is always concerned with improving the innate resistance of the individual and helping to build and strengthen vitality and inner strength. For this reason it has a major part to play in the treatment and prevention of all stress-related infection.

Character traits which aggravate the condition
Chronic stress is a powerful cause of recurrent infection in any part of the body, but particularly recurrent sinus, throat, or ear problems. The sustained build-up of stress drains energy reserves and depletes protective vital energy making you much more vulnerable to circulating viral or bacterial organisms. Unresolved grief, fear, anger or divorce, are the most common areas of tension which deplete natural resistance and cause an underlying weakening factor, which creates an ideal environment for infection to develop.

Practical steps to improve things
Keep your emotional life resilient and healthy, avoiding high intensity stress whenever possible. Try to find a more positive way of using your stress energy, and prevent it from damaging you. A healthy diet is always essential, high in natural vitamin C, also fresh air and regular daily exercise. If you live in an urban high density area, with pollution and poor air conditions, aim to spend some part of every weekend in a healthier area where you can relax and breathe cleaner air.

Remedies to consider:-

Antimon crud   Irritability is marked. The infections produce a discharge of pus. All symptoms are worse for heat or cold water.

Apis   There is a red swollen inflamed area, headache and vertigo. Tremor and extreme lassitude are other common symptoms.

Belladonna   For acute infections, with restlessness and pain, the affected area red, hot, and swollen.

Bryonia   Irritability is marked with anxiety about the future. There is marked thirst, the tongue coated white.

Hepar sulph   There is a combination of depression and irritability, with sharp splinter-like pains, worse for cold air, better for damp weather.

Pyrogenium   For an acute infection with restlessness, a high temperature and an offensive discharge. Burning pain in the infected areas is improved by active movement.

Sulphur   For chronic infections, with an offensive discharge and burning pain, worse for any form of heat.

INSECURITY

Lack of self-confidence can cause recurring doubts about ability, acceptance, being liked, or valued, undermining every aspect of life, and to some extent, every relationship. An underlying security problem also imposes uncertainty about work abilities, prospects for the future, being able to communicate and talk, really the ability to give out to others and to be understood.

The cause is often a psychological trauma in the early developmental years, often a subtle hurt, occurring at a time when the child, perhaps sensitive by nature, became insecure because he was made to feel so. The actual causes may be obscure, but some of the common factors include:- endless teasing, a jealous sibling, inability to get close enough to a remote father or mother who was distant, strict and a relentless disciplinarian, or sometimes uncaring.

Sometimes insecurity relates to an unhappy relationship with an older sibling who was endlessly competitive, demanding or aggressive; one who fought for all the attention, constantly naughty and punished, but later rewarded because the parents felt guilty. Perhaps the commonest causes of adult insecurity is parental divorce during childhood.

The break-up of the family is always a loss for the child and a deprivation to some degree. Often he is unable to relate to either a one-parent family or step-parent situation. Other common causes are physical or psychological trauma, abuse in one form or other during childhood, perhaps bullying at school or in the home, especially from a live-in adult partner.

Other causes which undermine the attainment of primary inner security are the loss of one or both parents in childhood, often from an illness or accident. This is always traumatic to security, especially the loss of a parent by suicide - in some cases it is the child who first discovers the body.

Homoeopathy helps build trust and security again, although inevitably it is a slow process. The remedies act by making contact with often painful areas of the original trauma, making the feelings (really blocked psychological energy), and memories more available for recall, helping to build solid bridges towards a more mature adult understanding. Homoeopathy also helps mature damaged or fragile aspects of the personality.

Character traits which aggravate the condition
The mind is often dominated by fear of failure, humiliation, rejection, weakness, often illness and sometimes just not coping. This may have become a way of life, or rather a defence against it, avoiding any deep or meaningful involvement which might have lead to vulnerability. Anxiety levels are usually far too high, anticipating a disaster around every corner.

Practical steps to improve things
Live much more in the present, rather than in the past or the future. Try to keep away from fear of anticipated disasters, as this will limit you in your contact with others, freedom to explore new situations, and more creative self-expressions. Practise going into unfamiliar situations, making new friends, and not crossing bridges before they occur. This will slowly strengthen you, but you will need to do so daily over a period of months.

Remedies to consider:-

Gelsemium

There is a fear of appearing in public, lack of energy and lassitude.

Ignatia

Insecurity is related to grief or loss with depression, tears, and anguish.

Lycopodium

Self-confidence is weak, with a constant desire to attract attention in some way. Often taking risks and being foolish. Fear of the future and lack of concentration.

Natrum mur

Never fully at ease in any new or social situations.

Pulsatilla

The insecurity is variable, like the emotions, due to avoidance of close relationships. There is a tendency to be dramatic, and on the fringe of most things in life.

Silicea

Insecurity is partly due to lack of drive, also lack of experience. There is a tendency to back-away from challenge or competitive situations.

Staphysagria

Irritability and oversensitivity to the opinions of others creates insecurity. Moods vary from irritability to sadness.

INSOMNIA

Sleep problems are among the commonest of stress symptoms and in many ways the most devastating. They contribute to exhaustion, lack of proper rest and the ability to switch off from problems for a few hours. Insomnia can manifest in several ways. One of the commonest is an inability to fall asleep, tossing and turning, restless and tired, desperate for sleep, but completely unable to drop off.

Stressful sleep is usually shallow, restless, frequently accompanied by disturbing dreams or nightmares. These may be particularly distressing and exhausting, often stimulated by violent or emotional television programmes or an overactive mind. The other common cause is too much coffee or tea during the day. In order to cure the problem, it is essential to break the caffeine habit, which is a social addiction and to avoid all late night television. Quiet music, a relaxation tape, or reading, are far better alternatives until the sleep habit is re-established.

Stress insomnia may manifest as an exhausting pattern of wakening in the early hours, sometimes only an hour or two after falling asleep. The person goes to bed and falls asleep perfectly easily, but is wide awake at one or two a.m. and totally unable to fall asleep again. He is usually under enormous psychological pressure and wakes worrying about the events of the day ahead; about not sleeping or coping, constantly getting up for drinks because his mouth is dry, or to empty the bladder. His mind may be stretched to breaking point by an excessive intake of thoughts and emotions, combined with only minimal rest.

A third type of insomnia occurs when there is a more depressive element to stress. Early morning wakening occurs after a relatively normal sleep; waking about 5.00 a.m. with a sense of anguish or foreboding fear, often 'butterflies' in the stomach, worrying about the day ahead, and what the demands will be. The early morning fears are usually about something seemingly quite trivial - taking down the net curtains, shopping, having the grandchildren for tea, a day-trip to the coast, but especially fearful of any kind of change. The sleep problem is usually compounded before Christmas, and at holiday times, birthdays, retirement, a house move, a change of job, and adding to the fund of problems to worry about.

Character traits which aggravate the condition

There is a tendency to be too tense, to carry work and worry home afterwards, not easily letting go of stress or the problems which occur, and too often anticipating difficulties in the future. All of this creates a tense, restless, worried personality and undermines relaxation.

Practical steps to improve things

Try to take more exercise during the day and stop worrying about what might happen. Enjoy life as it unfolds and see challenges and difficulties as steps leading to change and new opportunities. At the end of each day relax much more, aiming for a complete contrast at weekends and in the evening, a change of thinking and attitudes, as well as routine and habits. Avoid the habit of working and worrying, as it will drain you, make you over-tired, and build up tension which will then spill into sleep time. Regular relaxation periods during the day are helpful, also yoga or meditation.

121

Remedies to consider:-

Arsenicum   There is restless agitation, always feeling cold and irritable. There is obsessional neatness, with a tendency to wake after midnight.

Coffea   There is an inability to fall asleep, agitated, sweating, restless, often with palpitations or indigestion. Insomnia associated with a high caffeine intake.

Kali carb   There is a tendency to wake early, about 4-5.00 a.m. feeling anxious, depressed, fearful of the day ahead. Fatigue is marked.

Lycopodium   It is difficult to fall asleep because of an overactive, restless mind, usually worrying about the future and what might happen.

Natrum mur   Depression and sadness is marked, causing a restless sleep, with early morning waking.

Sepia   It is difficult to get to sleep as over-tired to the point of exhaustion. Backache, or dragging down abdominal or pelvic pains, are a constant irritating problem. These are worse at the end of the day.

IRRITABILITY AND VIOLENCE

Short-fuse irritability is a common stress symptom. In many instances it is caused by long-standing difficulties in verbal communication and social skills, with a poor control of emotion, frustration and aggression.

Irritability may be part of an underlying depressive mood and feelings of self-dissatisfaction, because standards are too high, or sometimes because of envy or jealousy problems, and feeling inadequate. Under the surface lies apprehension and weakness, anxiety about making a mistake, fear of rejection, or changing an established position which does not give fulfilment.
Fear of failure, not accepting chances or challenges when they occur, awareness of time passing, adds to the pressures. Irritability is increased by the need to do something quickly, or to make changes which are not easily defined. This may lead on to a moody dissatisfaction with life, and all too often, this is taken out on others. There is a tendency to be irritable with hesitancy, weakness or faults, with short-fuse temper outbursts at the wheel, in the supermarket, or when having to wait.

Violence is often an attempt to find a quick exit from a situation where the individual feels under pressure and one which he cannot easily discuss or negotiate. It tends to occur from lack of social experience, or weak verbal assertiveness skills. Sometimes the only way to express an opinion is in a violent, childish outburst reflecting poor controls, at the same time adding to underlying depression. Sometimes violence is more self-directed, leading to extremes of self-imposed pressures and demands, or accompanied by an excessive intake of alcohol, drugs, cigarettes, coffee or tea, which eventually undermine physical health. Uncontrollable anger may occur after an acute accident, such as loss or damage to a limb in a work-related trauma. After a head injury with concussion, the personality may change (as a result of the shock), and become far less understanding and tolerant. Accident proneness is common, and irritable, violent people tend to be their own worst enemy, each act of uncontrollable emotion leading to more depression and a lessening of confidence.

Character traits which aggravate the condition
Poor emotional controls, short-fuse excitement or irritability, fatigue, add to the alcohol-dependency. Impatience, anxiety, lack of confidence and poor verbal skills are other typical character traits.

Practical steps to improve things
Aim for greater relaxation in all aspects of life. Try to be more outgoing and spontaneous, less withdrawn and more positive overall. Gauge the areas where you feel most frustrated and irritated (often blocked by your own indecision or holding back), and clarify where and what you can change to improve the situation. Practise talking more, giving out more of yourself and avoid allowing emotions to build up to breaking point when you may loose control.

Aim to progress slowly and steadily in everything you do, and try to slow down and monitor your outbursts (of enthusiasm as well as your rage), yet not keeping yourself controlled or in check. Avoid floods of feelings and emotions which you cannot possibly control or discuss.

Remedies to consider:-

Aurum met There is violent short-fuse anger and irritability, with moods of suicidal depression.

Hepar sulph A remedy for hypersensitivity and irritability at the least provocation. Sharp splinter-like pains occur in the throat.

Hyoscyamus For irritability, associated with suspicion, and sudden mood swings with overactivity.

Nux vomica There is a combination of irritability with zealous enthusiasm for the underdog. Sudden spasms of violence and rage alternate with depression.

Lilium tig For irritability and impatience. Impulses to hit out alternate with depression.

Sepia Indicated for severe irritability associated with dragging down fatigue and pain, worse in the evening. Indifference to loved ones.

Tarentula For states of hysterical anguish with tears, irritability, and impulses to destructive behaviour.

IRRITABLE BOWEL SYNDROME

This is a common stress-related disorder of the lower colon and bowel region, often beginning in childhood or adolescence. It is associated with repressed (denied) emotional tensions, which find an exit through the lower colon and bowel. A build-up of emotional tension occurs, because of an underlying lack of confidence, fear, and self-doubts. There is an expectation of something going wrong, an event which cannot be coped with or embarrassing, showing you in a 'bad light' as weak or inadequate.

Emotional tension usually builds up before any social event, feeling trapped by something new or unusual but not necessarily unpleasant. A child may develop bowel problems before going to a party, an adult, when inviting the neighbours in for drinks, when visiting friends, going out for supper, or the theatre, a training day at work. Emotions accumulate because they cannot be fully expressed or shared, due to shame about the intensity of feelings and a sense of failure. The build-up of tension, spills over into the bowel area and becomes a habit over the years, an expression of the underlying anxiety.

The main symptoms which occur:- are a noisy rumbling abdomen, wind, difficulty in eating, loss of appetite, a dry mouth, colicky abdominal pain, or spasm, often a sense of discomfort felt along the descending colon (the left side of the lower abdomen). Diarrhoea is common, in a mild form as loose stools whenever there is an emotional pressure situation. The condition eventually occurs without any obvious trigger causing anxiety or tension and becomes chronic.

The condition often defies both diagnosis, or relief from conventional medicine, or any form of over-the-counter drugs. Over the years many methods of treatment may have been tried, but leading to only temporary or limited improvement.

Homoeopathy is helpful, because it acts upon the root cause within the personality, and helps mature areas of the personality dominated by infantile fear. There is a damaging tendency to undervalue yourself at the same time as over-valuing others.

Character traits which aggravate the condition
A tendency to withhold feelings and needs, not admitting to problems or talking about them fully and in depth. Controlling attitudes, irritability and frustration, are a frequent expression of the tensions felt. Lack of patience, and an inability to take a broad overview of life, makes it difficult to resolve the bowel problems.

Practical steps to improve things
Aim to be more open, easy, and relaxed. Don't worry so much about trifles or what might happen. Bowel irritability is often caused by too much emotion in the intestinal area, and this can be improved by talking and sharing more and making new friends. In all areas of social contact, aim for a more fluid and easy spontaneous approach to others.

Remedies to consider:-

Anacardium

There is indigestion with nausea and vomiting. All symptoms are worse for eating. Constipation is a problem, the bowels feel blocked as if by a 'plug'.

Arsenicum

Indicated for restless agitation with burning pains and diarrhoea. All symptoms are worse after midnight, and from cold.

Dioscorea

A remedy for shifting right-sided abdominal colicky pain, better for walking. Morning diarrhoea is a common problem.

Natrum sulph

For windy colic with a yellow watery diarrhoea, worse on waking. The mood is one of sadness, worse for music (which increases the depression).

Nux vomica

There are chronic problems of indigestion and constipation, associated with nausea or vomiting, spasms of colicky pain and severe irritability of mood.

Podophyllum

For problems of early morning diarrhoea with mucus. There is abdominal distention with a burning weakness, wind and belching.

ISOLATION AND WITHDRAWAL

Lack of confidence, often fear or mistrust, causes withdrawal into what is felt to be the only ultimate safe haven, namely the inner world of the self. Withdrawal is usually based on a distortion of others, lack of trust, and a tendency to fear other people's demands and the need to keep them at a 'safe' distance. If this is not achieved, it is often feared they will in some way attempt to limit or control you.

Beneath the fears is a feeling of vulnerability, doubts about self-confidence, being loved and accepted, leading to a sense of lonely isolation, an increasing tendency to live in an imaginative world of omnipotence and fantasy. But isolation is also a form of suffering, and a deprivation. The inner personality core does not easily mature and strengthen, or sustain confidence without emotional contact with others. If very severe, it may eventually lead to a schizoid or distorted view of life, in time to a possible break-down or schizophrenic illness.

The trigger factors leading to withdrawal may be a physical accident, the breakdown of a relationship, especially a recent separation or divorce. The sudden violent death of a much loved member of the family may leave feelings of total grief and devastation, where the only solution is felt to be total withdrawal as a reaction of shock and an expression of underlying depression and the mourning process.

The isolation may lead to physical deprivation as well as an emotional state, and this adds to weakness and fatigue, causing confusion.

Character traits which aggravate the condition

There is a tendency to isolate sensitive or vulnerable aspects of the self because of fear of getting hurt. Avoidance of others may occur, if they are seen as a potential threat or a danger. Self-denigratory attitudes are common, because suppressed feelings of rage, rejection and anger, are turned back upon the self and not given a more healthy outward acknowledgement and open expression.

Practical steps to improve things

Try to be more aware of your isolation and withdrawal from others. It is often a form of anger and rejection and may take time to perceive. Avoiding others usually aggravates any problems, and whenever possible this should be reduced or limited. Find friends and make new acquaintances with whom you can be more open. Try to be more caring, giving and spontaneous with others, including members of the family you are angry with. In relationships where you do not express yourself openly, try to see what your withdrawal means, the feelings concerned, and aim to become more involved, making more contacts with others of all ages.

Remedies to consider:-

Arsenicum   There is a rigid, obsessional, controlled approach to others, with depression, anxiety, also restlessness, and an inability to relax.

Ignatia   The isolation is linked to sadness and grief, associated with a recent loss or separation.

Natrum mur   A typical 'loner', close contact or consolation aggravates the sadness and depression. He never really feels at ease or relaxed with others.

Platina   Pride and arrogance are marked, inevitably leading to rejection, being hurt and feeling depressed or a failure. Others are kept at a distance.

Sepia   Contact with others leads to extremes of irritability and impatience. Many of the symptoms are related to severe dragging down tiredness.

Staphysagria   There are moods of severe irritability, always over-sensitive to the opinions of others.

JEALOUSY

Jealousy is present in us all at times, and is part of natural rivalry and territorial assertiveness. In part it has a preservative, self-defensive function and helps guard and protect a relationship; as well as playing a role in awareness, possessiveness, and security. It keeps a distance between other members of the same sex, who may try to 'poach' a partner, and maintains a healthy level of watching awareness and mistrust which can be useful, as long as it is not excessive. What matters always, is the degree and intensity of any jealousy present.

A little can be seen as a compliment to the partner, a confirmation of being loved, but in most cases jealousy is a destructive emotion, because it reveals an underlying sense of mistrust and insecurity. When severe, a jealous person can feel threatened by any person of the same sex, either in the present or the past, to the extent that a mother may feel jealous of her daughter, her youth and sexual appeal. Unless it is resolved within the couple or the family, it may lead to high levels of anguish, fear, mistrust, and suspicion. Often, it involves a child or close relative.

If jealousy is kept hidden and denied, or not openly discussed and talked about, it will tend to feed upon fear and fantasy. It then risks getting totally out of hand, destroying trust, and with it close relationships.

At times, it may lead to isolation, complete domination by fantasy, a nervous break-down, sometimes a severe psychological paranoid (persecutory) illness.

In the elderly, the problem may be associated with confusion, sometimes due to the side-effects of a prescribed drug, or because a senile degenerative state causes confusion. In many adult relationships, there is a lack of quite basic verbal communication and sharing, which may fuel insecurity and jealousy. In the majority of adult relationships, the couple need to find a better, more open way of communicating, including the sharing of fears and doubts, as well as affection, love and closeness.

The condition responds well to homoeopathy, which helps put the underlying fears and doubts into a more balanced perspective.

Character traits which aggravate the condition
There is a tendency to be mistrustful, to make comparisons, and there is a problem of basic security. In fantasy, others are felt to have too much power, malice, or to have designs on your partner, based on lack of confidence and fear.

Practical steps to improve things
Aim to be more outgoing, giving and spontaneous, less vulnerable, or influenced by others. Try to see your intrinsic strengths, and value yourself more. In this way you will eventually become more balanced in your perspectives and emotions, less vulnerable to suggestions or comments from others. Aim to live more in the present, to be more involved, interested in what is happening now, expressing what you feel, now in the present. Try to be less dominated by what others may be doing or thinking. Become more open and less concerned with plots and schemes. In that way, you will also feel more confident. Aim to trust others more.

133

Remedies to consider:-

Hyoscyamus   Impatience, jealousy and suspicion are associated with restless agitation and excitable mood swings. Quickly becomes irritable.

Ignatia   There are changeable moods, often involving jealousy or possessiveness, then becoming withdrawn, tearful, and sighing. The jealousy may be provoked by a recent shock or loss.

Lachesis   The tendency to jealousy and mistrust is associated with being lively and over-talkative. Moods are irritable and impatient, worse in the evening.

Nux vomica   There is jealousy with impatient irritability, over-sensitive to all impressions. He is typically thin, zealous, and too intense. Chronic indigestion and constipation are other problem areas.

Pulsatilla   Jealousy alternates with a variety of mood changes, from laughter to shyness, tears, indifference. All symptoms are worse for heat and better for fresh air. Thirst is absent.

LETHARGY AND TIREDNESS

Sluggish energy and extreme tiredness are frequent symptoms of stress and tension states, when restless anxiety has drained all energy reserves. There is sometimes a sense of feeling unreal, in a time-warp, an automaton figure, lacking initiative, as stress undermines drive. Fear of failure or disapproval is a common problem as others are perceived as powerful parental figures, arousing infantile feelings, guilt, and resentment.

Homoeopathy helps mature and integrate the personality, gradually creating a better internal balance and greater maturity. In this way, parental ties and identifications become less strong and there is greater tolerance and understanding of the different needs of each maturing person, bringing insight and growth.

Character traits which aggravate the condition
A tendency to be constantly anxious or guilty, especially fearing failure or criticism. There is a tendency to identify with the problems of others, taking on their burdens as well as your own, and worrying about them excessively.

Positive steps to improve things
Relax more, and be a support to yourself as much as to others. Try to get guilt feelings into perspective, clarify their origins when possible, and don't be a martyr to them. Don't pressure yourself, as this will cause exhaustion and leave you with insufficient reserves to cope with the day. Try to see yourself as you are today, not as a child. Keep your present aims and goals in focus, and move towards achieving them.

Remedies to consider:-

Arnica Feeling psychologically bruised, leading to exhaustion and anxiety. A very useful remedy after a nervous strain or emotional shock.

China Exhaustion is marked, often following an infection, with recurrent sweating, aching, and a slightly raised temperature. Fatigue follows a prolonged period of demanding work, i.e. nursing a sick relative.

Ferrum phos There is a tendency to nervous flushing of the face or neck, with exhaustion. All symptoms are worse in the evening, after a jolt, or any sudden movement.

Kali phos A useful remedy when there is a combination of irritability, and exhaustion with depression. The underlying cause is often a period of strain or high anxiety levels.

Nux moschata For drowsiness with exhaustion and changeable mood swings. A dry mouth and skin are indications for this remedy.

LIBIDO

Libido, or sexual drive and energy, is a major biological motivating force in every society. It is often depleted by stress, leading to almost total loss of interest, with closeness and affection also affected. The libidinal drive is closely related to confidence and relaxation and is always undermined by fear, anxiety, tension, anger or resentment, also by feelings of jealousy, loss of trust or closeness within the relationship.

Doubts about a commitment by the partner, feeling loved and valued, often relate back to childhood, when a combination of family and emotional problems undermined confidence.

The libidinal energy drive is a driving force for many activities throughout the day, but it can be undermined by tension, pressure, and an inability to relax. At times, libidinal interest is heightened by stress, especially during an overactive mood swing, with boundless energy, enthusiasm and optimism across a wide spectrum of ideas and drives, including excitement within the sexual sphere.

Libido may be heightened because it represents a flight from reality, denial of the need to resolve a problem area, a relationship difficulty, or an overwhelming need for reassurance and comfort. Heightening of libidinal drive is usually temporary and can easily swing back into fatigue and depression, because it is rooted in fear rather than genuine interest.

Character traits which aggravate the condition

There is inability to relax, or to ever fully let go, leading to fatigue, burn-out, irritability, a tendency to perfectionism, stress and tension. All may deplete the natural libidinal drives. Rigid attitudes and high expectations can also undermine sexual drive.

Practical steps to improve things

Relax more, and become more at ease with yourself, taking time off working and worrying. Accept the limitations as well as the gifts you have. Be kind to yourself, as well as to others. Don't drive yourself quite so much and trust your creative talents a little more.If there is a sexual problem, take more of an overview of the situation, and consider that lack of libidinal drive may relate to an unresolved problem within your relationship which you have not fully admitted. It is also caused by fear, apprehension and tiredness. Don't expect so much of yourself all the time and take the pressures off to allow your libidinal drive time to be re-established.

Above all, give yourself much more time for trust and confidence to be re-established, and for your energy reserves to be re-charged.

Remedies to consider:-

Agnus cast   There is a combination of chilly exhaustion with loss of libidinal interest.

Lycopodium   For high levels of restless anticipatory anxiety, and inability to relax. Fear and tension may undermine the libidinal drive and sexual confidence.

Natrum mur   The underlying problem is often a combination of depression with anxiety. Physical health is weak, with low body weight, the skin covered with sweat. There is a craving for salt. Closeness or consolation, tends to aggravate the problems. Never fully relaxed or at ease with others.

Sepia   There is a combination of exhaustion with dragging down low back and pelvic pain. All symptoms are worse in the evening. Fatigue and irritability undermine libidinal interest, and there is indifference to loved ones.

The specific drug in homoeopathic potency
When the problem relates to the side-effects of a particular drug.

LONELINESS

In an existential sense we are all ultimately alone, coming into the world alone, often suffering alone, and to some extent we must make our way and ultimately our exit alone. But this is a more healthy existential awareness of human pain and suffering, as well as human satisfactions and joy. Stress loneliness is mainly due to internal conflict, fear of strong dependency needs, often completely denying their strength, in case this leads to damaging rejection or pain.

Loneliness is a very common problem, often the result of stress, causing withdrawal and isolation from others. Despite the need for contact, and a meaningful happy relationship, the priority may be to avoid feeling vulnerable or being hurt.

Flight from others, can be both physical and psychological, keeping to a 'safe' distance, but always a lonely position, which usually means there is a conflict or split, with ambivalent feelings. The conflict may be related to the need for closer contact with others (hence the loneliness and feelings of need), contrasting with impulses to stay at uninvolved and at a safe distance.

The tendency to withdraw inwards often intensifies the feelings of loneliness, also the depression and frustration. Feeling isolated and trapped, with no possibility of allowing a close relationship to occur, adds to despair, anger and feelings of anguish.

Character traits which aggravate the condition
Insecurity, a tendency to develop infantile over-dependent relationships, lack of self-confidence.
There has often been a hurt or rejection during childhood, which lead to a tendency to keep at a distance from all close involvements. Because of the very strong feelings of need and closeness, this leads to feelings of vulnerability and fear of being hurt. This is shown in the character traits:- refusing to go to a party, as a child, and avoiding social engagements as an adult.

Practical steps to improve things
Everyone is lonely to some extent, even when they have a satisfying relationship. It is not possible to completely eradicate lonely feelings. But stress loneliness usually centres around feeling unhappy, sad and lonely when away from home or separate from the family or your partner. Try to value yourself more as a separate being. See yourself as a unique entity with a quality of life and try to value these gifts and qualities more. Loneliness is really another form of fear, often due to low self-esteem, an insufficient awareness of yourself as a separate and independent person.

Remedies to consider:-

Argentum nit   There is marked anxiety, fear, and insecurity. Time is felt to pass slowly. Impatient, all problems are worse for heat.

Kali carb   He is insecure, depressed, anxious, lonely and homesick. Never happy alone and rarely fully relaxed and at ease.

Lycopodium   Anticipation of failure causes anxiety and loss of confidence. Feels lonely, unless there is another person in the house, and then content to be in a room alone.

Phosphorus   For the person who dreads being alone, fearful always seeking company and reassurance. There is an excessive need for approval and to be liked.

Pulsatilla   This type of personality is constantly seeking company and reassurance, never happy alone but rarely contented when in company either. Always changeable and unpredictable. Moody, tearful, emotional outbursts are common.

142

MASTURBATION - anxiety or guilt feelings

Self-induced sexual satisfaction is perfectly normal human behaviour and usually present from infancy in both boys and girls. It should be regarded as a comfort and an outlet in times of tension or anxiety, often a way of finding relief from accumulated sexual frustration.

Masturbation in itself is not a problem, only if it becomes an end in itself, an obsessional preoccupation, with avoidance of others, does treatment need to be considered.

Masturbation is an outlet for accumulated sexual thoughts of all types. These are often about infantile control, power over others (ultimately the parents), and usually omnipotent and aggressive (but sometimes passive), sadistic fantasies. Problems occur because of the intensity of feelings which the fantasies conjure up, leading to misplaced guilt, anxiety, or shyness. There may be a split between 'bad' sexual feelings (because of the pleasure associated with the fantasies), and 'good' sexual fantasies (which match the parental or family model). These are more concerned with the socially acceptable feelings of love, sharing, having children, building a home, and family life.

As masturbation is more openly discussed and talked about, it is less of a taboo subject and much of the guilt and excessive anxiety has lessened. Where there is, or has been, exposure to a very strict, closed-in and oppressive family situation with rigid attitudes and puritanical values, then all forms of sexuality may be seen as undesirable and become linked to guilt, anxiety, fear, and timidity.

Man is a highly complex animal with powerful primitive drives and needs, and it is important to be able to accept, love, and understand, all aspects of yourself, including the sexual or sadistic fantasies which occur as well as the most tender and sublime feelings. Both accompany all phases of human growth and development. We are most aware of these two sides of man, our complex sexual feelings, and often ambivalence, in dreams.

Homoeopathy helps release feelings of repressed rage, anger, resentment, misunderstandings into the light of day, and makes for a healthier integration of a wide range of feelings and fantasy, weaving them into a more tolerant mature totality.

Character traits which aggravate the condition
There is a tendency to withdraw, to become isolated from others, relying too much on fantasy life and not enough on a reality relationship. There has often been a trauma to healthy normal development because of rejection, or overwhelming fear and anger.

Practical steps to improve things
Try to be more accepting of all aspects of yourself, including your sexual drive, interests and fantasies. See masturbation as an expression of a normal, biological and basic thrust (or force), for survival of the human race. Aim to be less self-critical and more tolerant of the many different aspects of yourself. At the same time, work towards giving out more, and moving towards others. Avoid obsessional thinking and rigid patterns of behaviour, as these can easily become engrained and difficult to alter. Consider relaxation, yoga, or meditation as helpful resources.

Remedies to consider:-

Hyoscyamus　　　There is a tendency to be both irritable and in a 'high' mood of elation. Although talkative and easily excitable, tends to lack confidence, and often suspicious of other people and their motives.

Lycopodium　　　There may be a problem of compulsory masturbation because of high anxiety levels. Lack of confidence and fear of the future increases anxiety levels. Lives in a fantasy world where sexuality is acted-out, but never expressed in reality.

Natrum mur　　　Moods of depression with tearful anxiety are common. The libidinal drive is often low. Masturbation may be used to bolster confidence, and as an outlet for failure to establish a close viable relationship.

Phosphorus　　　Anxiety levels are high, with over-sensitivity and enormous needs for acceptance and approval.

NAIL-BITING

This is often a symptom of repressed aggression, as the symbolic human claws of the body are gnawed away, at times of tension, anxiety, or fear. It is a common symptom of a repressed personality, dominated by the need to control criticism, anger, or anything that may cause rejection or disapproval. At times the human animal can be both predatory and aggressive. This is common in children, but also occurs in adults, and if these energies are totally denied without an alternative outlet, their drive is directed inwards to gnaw away at the self,with doubts and fears. This leads to a distortion of personality, creating a superficially 'good' or 'nice' conforming individual, but really someone who is only 'half a person', driven by fear of failure, disapproval, and non-acceptance. Nail biting often reflects a damaged personality, usually shy or inhibited, unable to express the fullness of his individuality. Homoeopathy helps unblock some of the repressed aggression, enabling it to be seen as less omnipotent or destructive, more acceptable and healthy.

Character traits which aggravate the condition
There is a tendency to be too controlled, too much in charge of feelings and reactions, to the detriment of spontaneity with others. Shyness, sensitivity, fear of others, undermines confidence.

Practical steps to improve things
Aim to more spontaneously express your thoughts and feelings as they occur. Avoid taking up a 'shy' position, where you are 'good' and conforming, when really your true position is much more controversial. Be more open with your feelings, with less guilt, and less apologetic.

Remedies to consider:-

Euphrasia   There are irritable and fretful moods, and these are reflected in the nail-biting. Always feels better in the fresh air.

Ledum   For tense and irritable moods, preferring to be alone. He is often critical of others, and frequently alcohol is taken to excess.

Nux vomica   Most emotions are too intense and excessive. Passionate ideals and involvements dominate much of the thinking.

Phosphorus   The habit is due to tension and fear, especially of being ignored or not approved of. Anxiety levels are high, with low self-confidence. Tends to flush-up easily.

Pulsatilla   All symptoms are variable, like the moods, from despair and tearful anguish, to dramatic gestures and laughter. Basic self-confidence is weak, and this often causes the tension symptoms.

Silicea   For the thin, sweating, anxious, sensitive person, who lacks drive, perseverance, and confidence.

NECK TENSION PROBLEMS

The neck is a common area of tension because it controls the head, movement of the face and eyes, and has a special role in unconscious body language and the expressions of the individual. It is a common area to be affected, especially with pain (from accumulated stress) and tension (due to muscular spasm), often made worse by bad posture, lack of relaxation, and any situation of irritability or frustration. In particular, the sternomastoid muscles go into spasm and become tight and hard, the head rigid and tense, and problems may occur in other areas of the body.

Any tendency to be stiff and rigid psychologically, tends to worsen neck tension. This is likely to occur where there is an obsessional type of temperament, dominated by rigid rules with overstrict controls and predictable attitudes, lack of spontaneity, and a tight unbending approach to life.

Homoeopathy helps by bringing any stress tensions, and the underlying psychological factors, to the surface.

Character traits which aggravate the condition
There is a tendency to withhold feelings, with a tight hold on emotions and spontaneity. Too much priority is given to obsessional neatness and order.

Practical steps to improve things
Try to spot the main times when the neck tension occurs and any trigger factors, particularly of an emotional kind which cause discomfort or pain. Practise regular relaxation exercises of the neck areas. Massage supports the remedies, and is recommended.

Remedies to consider:-

Arnica The neck feels bruised and tender, often the result of an emotional shock or trauma.

Baryta carb A useful remedy for painful neck problems, associated with fatigue, tension, and stress, also weakness after an illness or operation.

Causticum The personality is always very sympathetic and easily moved, but lacking confidence and is often depressed. There is stiffness of the neck area with restlessness and intermittent pain. All symptoms are improved by damp, moist conditions and heat.

Nux vomica The neck problem is associated with irritability and spasms of tension. All symptoms are worse for noise, bright lights, and strong odours. Impatient, and always too tense.

Rhus tox The neck tension is better for warmth and movement, worse for cold, inactivity, and on waking.

NIGHTMARES

Nightmares are really anxiety dreams, interfering with sleep, and associated with a pressurised overloaded mind. They represent a failure of the dream mechanism, which is essentially there to protect and preserve sleep, at the same time allowing the mind to continue to function. Nightmares occur from childhood onwards. They usually contain a wish-fulfilment or a primitive aggressive theme, often of a sadistic nature, for example, being attacked or chased, unable to escape some form of persecution. The sense of the nightmare is not always clear, but it often represents feelings of fear, becoming trapped, or blocked by a frightening situation, with feelings of rage and anger. An isolated nightmare may be triggered by an excess of food or alcohol, and is of no special significance, although the emotions felt at the time, often mirror undeclared and buried aspects of the self which have never been integrated. If nightmares become recurrent, interfere with sleep, or cause fear, look at, and try to understand the underlying cause.

Character traits which aggravate the condition
There is a tendency to hold feelings in, too timid or fearful, with denial of anger or aggression.

Practical steps to improve things
Aim to be more open with your feelings. Talk more about any fears or anxieties with your partner, a friend or the family. Don't keep emotions buried and under the surface. Share more of **you** and try to make your goals a reality. Be more adventurous and daring. Don't hold back on life, or yourself.

Remedies to consider:-

Belladonna
For agitated restless sleep with frightening dreams of violence, being followed, or fire. The face is usually red and hot. Sweating occurs in bed.

China
The nightmares cause waking, associated with a powerful feeling of weakness and oppression.

Hyoscyamus
Insomnia, unable to fall asleep as the mind is overactive. Very jerky and restless, the dreams frightening, violent and attacking.

Nux vomica
The problem is associated with indigestion, and intense violent dreams.

Stramonium
The sleep is disturbed by vivid dreams of the past, or frightening strange dreams. Waking with a cry or a scream. There is usually extreme restlessness.

Sulphur
Palpitations occur, feeling restless and burning hot in bed.

OBESITY

This is often the outcome of an underlying stress problem, although the causes are not always realised at the time. Emotional pressures, and often feelings of frustration or depression are not openly admitted. There is a destructive tendency to compensate for unhappiness, needs for closeness and affection, by over-eating, often between meals. Savoury, or high-calorie sweet foods, such as ice cream, cake, or chocolate, (which are high in calories), are indulged in.

Often the problem has existed for several years, sometimes since childhood. Many parents deal with tensions and problems in the home by 'rewarding' passivity and a non-challenge with food, sometimes a meal, which is high in calories. Many mothers control the cries or questions of a demanding child, by initially giving him a dummy, and later a sweet if he is 'good'. Food may be given to a child or teenager for not making 'trouble' by raising something awkward which worries the child, but the mother or parent feels unable to face up to.

It is not uncommon for the whole family to be overweight as the mother deals with her husband in the same way as the children, at the same time denying her own needs for more positive closeness, appreciation, and time. Obesity is frequently the outcome of this repression of all serious or controversial emotional issues. Lack of regular exercise, a high calorie diet, usually rich in saturated fats and cholesterol, adds to the general problem.

The entire family may become more prone to cardio-vascular disease, the possible early development of arteriosclerosis (hardening of the arteries), high blood-pressure, a 'stroke', or heart attack.

This kind of controlled approach to family problems is dangerous, and encouraged by a rigid or repressive upbringing and education. It is perpetuated by the model of the parents, where all of life is happy and there are no 'problems' (because they are denied). The emphasis is on a 'bonny' fat baby and child, with lovely round cheeks. The obesity problem may however put the health of the family at risk, sometimes an entire community, when it is official policy to encourage oral (eating) escapism and denial, rather than dialogue.

Character traits which aggravate the condition
There is a tendency to deny or repress all emotional problems, and to avoid talking them through within the family. Frustration and tension is denied by escaping into fantasy, usually too much television, and dealing with stress by eating, smoking, chewing and alcohol.

Practical steps to improve things
Avoid dieting or fasting. Aim to eat sensibly and healthily, with a calorie-controlled way of eating which you can enjoy and feel comfortable with. For greater psychological health, talk more about your needs and feelings, as soon as you are aware of them. If you feel exasperated, frustrated, or angry, then say so, without trying to be polite, or someone other than yourself. You can apologise later. Avoid snack eating, particularly at times of stress or tension. Regular exercise will help to tone up your muscles, but is unlikely to lead to a substantial weight loss.

153

Remedies to consider:-

Calcarea

Fearful and depressed, with obsessional tendencies. He is pale, always cold, covered in sweat, particularly around the head. There is a lack of energy and drive, with sour-tasting indigestion problems. Recurrent infections are common.

Kali carb

Weakness with chronic lethargy and exhaustion are indications for the remedy. He is often moody, either anxious or depressed. Lacking confidence, he feels insecure if alone in the house. There is a tendency to wake early, about 3-5.00 a.m. feeling anxious and tense with a sense of anguish about the day ahead.

Sulphur

There is a tendency to eat constantly without ever feeling full or satisfied. Energy and drive are lacking, but talking and expounding ideas is endless. None of them come to fruition. Chronic morning diarrhoea (which is offensive), indigestion problems with wind and flatulence. He feels worse from all forms of heat.

OBSESSIONS

Obsessional attitudes are a common part of many stress problems:- the emphasis on exaggerated self-control, manipulation of others, magical thinking, fear of change, and vulnerability.

The obsessional attitude is ritualistic, with a complex assortment of repetitive thoughts, omnipotent actions, and superstitious avoidances. There is an exaggerated fear of causing damage, either in the present or the past by a trivial action, and conviction that if the obsessional ritual is not followed to the letter, it will provoke a major catastrophe. The disaster is usually the loss of someone who is particularly needed and cared about. There may have been a major psychological trauma in early infancy, at a time when omnipotent thinking was normal for the particular stage of development, and causing damage to trust and confidence.

Homoeopathy helps soften the rigid thought patterns, helping to integrate any psychological damage which occurred into a wider, more mature understanding, and bringing balance, calm and relaxation.

Character traits which aggravate the condition
There is a controlled, rigid, neat approach to every aspect of life, which is based on magical thinking, and avoidance of the real issues which exist.

Practical steps to improve things
Try to be more easy and open with others and events as they occur. Especially avoid the habit of trying to ward off a negative fate by obsessional patterns, as this reinforces infantile omnipotent ways of thinking.

Remedies to consider:-

Arsenicum
There is marked obsessional neatness and controlling behaviour over every aspect of life. He is always exhausted, thin, and avoiding social contact with others. Burning indigestion pains are common. All symptoms are worse after midnight.

Calcarea
A remedy for obsessional thinking and rigid repetitive attitudes, always chilly, and often overweight. The skin sweats profusely, especially on the head at night making the pillow damp. He is anxious, obstinate, irritable, lacking confidence. There is a tendency to avoid others. Energy and drive are minimal, with constant complaints of exhaustion.

Natrum mur
A very useful remedy for a controlled personality with aversion to close contact with others. Worse for sympathy or consolation. Depression with tearful anxiety is marked. He is usually thin and covered in sweat, weak with no energy reserves. Ideas and thought patterns, like the body, are narrow, tight, and rigid.

156

PALPITATIONS AND PULSE IRREGULARITY

In health we are unaware of the heart beating, except after exercise, an abnormal effort, or strain. Because of too much tension or anxiety, there is an overspill of emotions into the conducting pathways of the heart. These may then become sensitized by the abnormal emotional energy current relayed through them causing a variety of cardiac irregularities. The commonest is an extra (early) heart beat followed by a compensatory pause, which may seem endless, as if the heart will never re-start. Other stress cardiac symptoms are:- a feeling of fullness in the chest; a pressure sensation as if the heart could burst; localised needle-sharp pains, or tenderness of the sternum (anterior chest wall) region; a vague sense of the heart moving or fluttering leading to discomfort; pressure or heat in the upper back or between the shoulder blades. This is due to referred discomfort because of the changes in cardiac rhythm. Shortness of breath or sighing breathing may occur in any stress situation. Symptoms are always aggravated by a high caffeine intake, especially excesses of coffee or tea. These should be strictly avoided.

Character traits which aggravate the condition
Oversensitivity and fear are the major features which cause the condition to develop, combined with shyness and a tendency to deny, or push down all emotional issues. Fussy perfectionism is often present.

Practical steps to improve things
Avoid anxiety taking you over, and keep emotional issues in balance by discussing them early with your partner. Try to avoid being a perfectionist. This makes you more vulnerable to a panic or fear reaction.

Remedies to consider:-

Calcarea   For obesity with a chilly
                    exhaustion, associated with
                    marked lack of confidence and
                    fear of close social contacts. The
                    palpitations are related to the
                    general state of weakness and
                    tension.

Convallaria   A very useful heart remedy. The
                    palpitations are often associated
                    with smoking, and nicotine-
                    induced. Feels worse for moderate
                    exercise.

Crataegus   A heart tonic, for strained or weak
                    cardiac conditions, with
                    irregularity of the heart beat,
                    raised blood-pressure and
                    arteriosclerosis. Exhaustion is
                    marked, with shortness of breath
                    on effort.

Natrum mur   Palpitations and extra heart beats
                    occur, with a rapid pulse. The
                    heart problem is often associated
                    with depression and a stress
                    tension state. Salt is usually
                    craved and taken to excess.

Spigelia   A useful remedy for pounding
                    palpitations, with fullness of the
                    chest. Shortness of breath, better
                    for sips of warm water.

PEPTIC ULCER

Stress often plays a major role in either gastric or duodenal (peptic) ulcer problems. This is because any unexpressed or strong emotional feelings inevitably react upon the stomach and upper intestinal regions. Usually this will only cause damage if the stress tensions are sustained over a period of months or years.

But powerful emotions always have some effect upon the digestive tube, causing dilatation of blood vessels within the mucosal lining area, and an increase of acid secretions.

Most manifestations of stress indigestion tend to become recurrent problems, especially symptoms of:- constant nausea, pain, fullness discomfort, flatulence, gassy eruptions of wind, heartburn, acidity, and sometimes insomnia due to discomfort from the pain. A peptic ulcer usually follows a prolonged period of stress, either at work, or in the home. Typical examples include:- being made redundant, failing to get promotion, the break-up of an engagement or marriage, the pain and hurt of a divorce, anger and resentment about a particular issue, including a recent trauma such as a loss, a violent traffic accident, or an assault involving a close member of the family.

In some cases, there is no obvious trauma or 'cause', and the ulcer seems the result of a temperament that worries, and sees fears or dangers whenever a decision has to be made, or a change is necessary.

A peptic ulcer can also occur as the side-effect of various prescribed over-the-counter drugs, especially analgesics or pain killers containing aspirin, also Brufen (Ibuprofen).

Homoeopathy helps relieve the symptoms and cure the condition. It also supports a healthier, more balanced approach to any stress problems which are undermining harmony, or provoking tension. If there is a physical blockage, such as scar tissue or narrowing of the stomach or intestine, this may require surgical treatment before the full benefits of homoeopathy can be felt.

Character traits which aggravate the condition
A tendency to worry excessively rather than taking the necessary steps to resolve a particular problem. Lack of social confidence leads to isolation, an impoverished emotional life, and lack of confidence. There is a tendency to be a perfectionist. Feelings and emotions are pushed down or denied, rather than discussed in an easy open way.

Practical steps to improve things
Try to be more outward looking, less self-critical, and easier with yourself, also less critical of others. Share your feelings, and always express them spontaneously. Especially avoid long periods of partially suppressed anger, jealousy, or envy. If you feel any of these, or other strong emotions, discuss them with the people concerned, as soon as you experience the feelings. Try to broaden and vary your interests. Avoid becoming too narrow in your interests and contacts. Regular periods of relaxation help to ease the condition, also consider yoga or meditation. Appreciate more what you have, rather than resenting what you don't have.

Remedies to consider:-

Hydrastis There is a sinking weakness in the stomach area with a soreness or dull pain, wind, and flatulence. A bitter taste in the mouth is characteristic.

Kali bich The stomach is inflamed, and feels swollen with severe burning pain, often vomiting. All symptoms are worse for wearing tight clothing or any pressure, better for eating. There is a dislike of meat.

Nux vomica Irritability is marked with a zealous short-fuse temperament. Everything is rushed, and too intense. Only minimal time is given to eating and digesting a meal. Nausea and vomiting may occur, also chronic constipation.

Ornithogalum There is weakness with depression, the chest and upper abdomen tight and distended. Haemorrhage may occur as a 'coffee-ground' vomit, or passing a black and tarry stool.

Phosphorus Loss of appetite occurs with nausea or vomiting, also heart-burn and flatulence. Pain is better for ice-cold food or drinks.

161

PHOBIA

This is one of the commonest symptoms of stress pressure. The person is dominated by unreasonable and irrational fears, always feeling unsafe and vulnerable. Typical fears include:- being alone in the house; fear of vomiting; choking, diarrhoea or fainting; also anxiety when eating in public; using a lift or escalator; fear of flying; driving on motorways or long distances, when it would be impossible to return home quickly.

Phobias tend to be rigid control systems, promoting the *status quo*, the known and familiar, in any type of situation. Ultimately they are a defence against childish emotions, especially feeling vulnerable, insignificant, and small. To this extent they are infantile and have their roots in infantile anxieties. The phobic problem often originates at an early age, the result of an acute fear situation, perhaps going into hospital, being separated from the parents, being abused or bullied, evacuated, or any break-up of the family. Any form of stress in the present may reactivate these early anxieties.

Character traits which aggravate the condition
There is a rigid omnipotent approach to life, often based on ritual and obsessional patterns. All emotions tend to be over-controlled and avoided, because it is feared their effect on others will be overwhelming.

Practical steps to improve things
Aim to limit the power of any rituals by slowly reducing their frequency and substituting more open spontaneous behaviour. Discuss your phobias openly with others. This helps to reduce their omnipotence, and the damage to your psychological freedom.

Remedies to consider:-

Argentum nitricum Anxiety and fear are marked, especially concerned with fear of flying or speaking in public. Hypochondriacal fears cause anxiety about health. Fatigue and exhaustion are worse in the late morning, just before noon.

Arsenicum Weakness and fear are characteristic of the problems, always cold and craving heat in any form. There are many obsessional fears, especially of the illness, death, losing control or becoming violent. All the symptoms are worse in the early hours, after midnight.

Calcarea Always feeling cold, fearful, and exhausted, obstinate. Fear of noise, other people, and illness.

Gelsemium A useful remedy for mild but dramatic phobic problems. Much of the fear links to public appearances, for example examination nerves, giving a sermon or a public talk.

Natrum mur Depression with tearful anxiety and fear. Avoids contact with others. He feels chilly, weak and exhausted.

PREMATURE EJACULATION

This is a distressing male problem, with a tendency to premature orgasm from any form of intimate caressing, or almost immediately after penetration. The man is usually unsure of himself, anxious and tense, especially with a new partner, or when he feels under pressure to perform or to prove himself. He may find it difficult to ever relax completely, to feel free to discuss feelings in depth, and fears loss of control.

When problems occur, the man may have been anxious about his performance over a period of several months, having previously experienced a precipitate orgasm. There is usually a great deal of intense emotion; feeling rushed, under pressure, often angry or irritable. He has a tendency to rush everything, to be quick or short-fuse in almost every situation in life, anticipating problems, and rarely pacing himself so that he can feel more confident and relaxed, and under less pressure.

Character traits which aggravate the problem
A tendency to rush at everything, irritable and always under pressure, most of which is self-created. Confidence with women is low because of fear, and lack of social experience with the opposite sex.

Practical steps to improve things
Reduce pressure in all areas, and aim to be more at ease with both men and women. Build-up more social confidence, before creating a pressurised intimate situation you are unsure of. Avoid attempting intercourse until you feel relaxed and confident. Spend more time holding and caressing. Share feelings and needs, giving yourself more time in all aspects of life.

Remedies to consider:-

Agnus cast   A useful remedy when there is a reduced sexual drive and low vitality, with weakness and depression.

Borax   Ejaculation is rapid, followed by feelings of continual irritation within the penis.

Fluoricum ac   For excessive sexual excitement with poor controls. The scrotal sac is often swollen.

Kali phos   There is a combination of weakness and exhaustion combined with quickness, and a flashing intensity of feelings.

Lycopodium   Anxiety and tension occurs, with lack of self-confidence. The sexual problem is part of a general tendency to be rushed, too quick and premature in every aspect of life.

Picricum ac   There is weakness of the sexual urge, with a rapid involuntary emission, followed by exhaustion.

PUBLIC SPEAKING ANXIETY

This is a common stress problem and one which can create terrors in an otherwise confident male or female. There may be total confidence in all other social areas, but the thought of speaking out in public, getting up to say something in a crowded meeting, at a wedding, in a work or large group situation, strikes pangs of panic, and terror. Loss of confidence may similarly occur in any situation where you feel on display, or a critical judgment may be made.

Fears vary with the individual, but include:- drying up, loss of voice, becoming high-pitched, or the voice weak, feeling tongue-tied, confused, over anxious, red or sweating. Others develop a tremor, feel faint or nauseated in a public situation.

The problem often reflects psychological immaturity, a blockage to confidence and personality growth often stemming from childhood. There may be a tendency to distort others, to see them in an inflated or over-valued way, including seeing an audience as critical or superior. In some ways, this repeats a childish position, the audience seen as the parents or authority figures, who are there to watch, but take on a critical superior role. There may be too much emphasis on comparison with others, which is damaging to confidence and partly based on unresolved childhood jealousy or envy, usually involving a parent or sibling.

The problem may also relate to inexperience in large group situations, always ill at ease with others because as a child you had little, or no experience of talking and playing in groups with siblings, or other children of your own age. Talking loudly or spontaneously may have been frowned upon, threatened with punishment, disapproval, laughter, which undermined confidence at the time. Infantile fears of humiliation may still be present years later, and cause the adult to experience anxiety and to take flight.

This type of problem responds well to homoeopathy, helping to build-up and mature weak areas of the personality, supporting greater self-confidence and trust.

Character traits which aggravate the condition
Shyness, a tendency to overvalue others, to be self-critical and reluctant to compete or communicate openly. The major problem is fear of humiliation or loss of face, where others are seen as a powerful threat. This is usually based on negative infantile experience and sometimes a severe trauma.

Practical steps to improve things
Avoid any tendency to withdraw when asked to speak in public. This will further undermine confidence and self-trust. Make a point of publicly saying what you feel, as and when you feel it. Try to let your individuality sing out to others in a voice which can be heard without fear of disapproval. Practise talking in small groups, socially and in public about topics which interest you and where you are knowledgeable. Ask questions in meetings and try to do so regularly. Avoid keeping to the periphery of a group or life, or taking a vague, shadowy position on a topic. If you don't know, say so firmly. If you have an opinion, let it out clearly and be prepared to defend it.

Remedies to consider:-

Argentum nit   There is fear, apprehension, lack of self confidence and intolerance of heat. All the anxieties are worse in a public situation and for heat. Assertiveness is low.

Gelsemium   There is a variable, hysterical depression, with tension, often excessive anxiety and lethargy.

Lycopodium   Fear, tension, and lack of confidence, causes the panic attack. He is always too tense and striving to be accepted.

Pulsatilla   Every public speech is turned into a dramatic performance, felt to be a disaster, although in reality a success. Tears are followed by extremes of emotion, and always feeling worse from heat.

Silicea   Chilly, thin, lacking in drive and self-confidence. Always fears a rejection. Under pressure, there is a tendency to sweat profusely.

SEXUAL FEARS AND ANXIETIES

These are commonplace, occurring in both sexes from the early teens onwards. A wide variety of problems occur, nearly always based on distortion and faulty assumptions, shyness and fear, lack of confidence, immaturity, lack of experience, or previous damage.

A combination of tension, spasm and withdrawal, due to anxiety, is responsible for failing to respond immediately, or perform on demand. This creates a variety of stress-related problems. These include weakness of the sexual drive, or it may be felt to be uncontrollable and overwhelming, taking you over, obvious and noticeable to everyone.

Masturbation anxieties are a common source of the problems (see section, page 144). There may also be fear of the opposite sex, based on early infantile sexual fantasies:- being swallowed up, taken over, treated violently, raped, hurt or damaged in a vague but terrifying and paralysing way. There is often fear of the unknown, what the sexual act may be, rather than what it actually is, thinking about it in isolation from an actual relationship, failing to see intercourse as a highly individual creative act, uniting love and affection with instinctual and biological needs.

Sexual anxieties are common to everyone. If the natural apprehension is fed and encouraged by fantasy, lack of contact with the opposite sex, failure to verbalise, share and discuss what is feared, then problems may occur.

Many sexual fears are the result of upbringing as well as sensitivity and could be prevented if there was a more open healthier attitude within the family. Children should be encouraged to talk to their parents much more about sex and their sexual anxieties. Parents should answer questions directly and honestly when asked, without embarrassment, keeping the language to a level which the child can understand. They need not elaborate beyond the boundaries of the particular query or question, as a healthy child will always ask what he is unsure of and needs to know. Teenagers should also have more opportunity to talk about every aspect of sex within the family, because this is one of their major preoccupations, as the libidinal motor begins to be activated. Girls should be informed about their periods, preferably before the event, and teenagers should not only learn about sex from their peers, or in the playground, but also from within their family.

Character traits which aggravate the condition

There is a tendency to be remote from others, especially contact with the opposite sex during the early formative years. Emotions are kept buried, including sexual curiosity, anger, jealousy, the need for understanding and affection. Shyness, greatly increases the problems.

Practical steps to improve things

The best way to lessen anxiety, is to stimulate contacts and discussions, which will improve your levels of confidence and maturity. Aim for a very varied social contact with others, friendships with both sexes and of all ages. Try to give and participate more in all of these. Discuss any sexual fears or problems within your relationship as soon as you are aware of a difficulty and avoid keeping it to yourself as a dark secret. Talk more freely to your partner, sharing thoughts and feelings, including your sexual fantasies.

Remedies to consider:-

Argentum nit   A remedy for nervous fears and hypochondriacal attitudes. Fear of failure. All problems are worse from heat.

Cicuta virosa   There is anxiety with sweating, tremor, and lack of confidence. A tendency to be very fearful and imaginative.

Gelsemium   Sadness, depression and lethargy are typical indications for this remedy. Vaginismus due to spasm may occur in females, impotency in males. Everything is dramatised, and it is never easy to be natural and relaxed.

Graphites   Indicated for timid, indecisive, fidgety anxiety, fearing failure because of a basic lack of self-confidence.

Pulsatilla   Everything is variable, with excessive emotions, tears, and intolerance of heat.

Silicea   For timidity and weakness, with a constant need for reassurance. Resistance to fatigue is low, also drive and determination.

171

SHYNESS

A shy person is nearly always stressed, reflecting high levels of anxiety, intense self-consciousness, fear and anxiety about meeting others, often the need to run away from situations where he lacks confidence. Shyness can be a very painful and distressing condition which begins in childhood and persists throughout the teens into adult life. It is a limiting factor as far as contact with others is concerned, because it acts as a barrier to closeness, social comfort and spontaneous free-expression.

Anger is never far from the surface and leads to the quick peevish temperament of the shy person, although rarely admitted and often kept hidden from others until it boils over. Most anger is directed inwards, usually in a self-critical way. Occasionally, a younger more dependent sibling, can be at the receiving end of a lot of anger or bullying.

Much of the shyness is related to repressed sexual interests and drive, which are felt to be unacceptable, and kept private or hidden. This is often due to the infantile aspects of the sexual drives, and because sexual interest or looking is associated with guilt.

Shyness is usually associated with feelings of guilt, shame, or self-consciousness. The problem also reflects need for attention and to be noticed, although, consciously this is the last thing in the world you would wish for. Usually there is a combination of contrasting wishes:- to be in the limelight, seen and approved of, at the same time a wish to be on the edge, and just one of the group.

Once shyness can be accepted as something more ordinary and 'normal', that everyone is a little shy, especially in new situations, then the shyness problem and any associated sexual fantasies can be more openly admitted and understood.

Character traits which aggravate the condition
There is a tendency to withdraw and to hide, yet in some way always managing to inevitably draw attention to yourself, often in an awkward, embarrassing or unwelcome way.

Practical steps to improve things
Aim always to be as easy and spontaneous as you can with others. Make contact with any group of people you want to be with, including young people of the opposite sex, and those you judge to be authoritarian (really parental), success figures. Increase your contact with others in a wide variety of social situations, being open and spontaneous with them. If you are feeling particularly shy, then admit it or make a joke or talking point around shyness feelings. Avoid hiding yourself away or becoming involved with secret fantasies which you are not discussing with your partner or family. Also see the section on Blushing (page 52).

Remedies to consider:-

Ambra grisea   Feels anxious, sad, or irritable,
especially in the evening, the
mind in a dream-like state. Fear
of close contact with others.

Natrum mur   Shyness is part of an overall
pattern of lack of confidence, fear
and often tearful depression. All
social contacts are a source of
tension and anxiety and he is
never either natural or relaxed.
Always worse for sympathy or
consolation. Weak, thin, and
exhausted, he is a typical loner.

Lycopodium   A major problem is impulsiveness
and anticipatory anxiety. Too
quick in every situation in life.
There is a combination of
insecurity and over-intense
reactions which cause instability.

Pulsatilla   Shyness is marked, with mood
swings, varying from tearful
depression to anger or laughter.
All contacts tend to be superficial,
over-emotional, or dramatised.
The discomfort is always worse in
a hot or stuffy room.

174

SLEEPWALKING AND SLEEP TALKING

Sleepwalking is a common problem of sensitive nervous children, also adolescents, and less often in adults. At the time, there is a dissociated state of mind. The child, while still sleeping deeply, gets up for a drink or food, to go downstairs, into the kitchen or another room, sometimes silently, or saying an unintelligible word or two and then returning to bed. He is not usually at risk or accident-prone at this time, and all movements are slow, controlled and deliberate. It is not usually related to an underlying physical or neurological condition, such as epilepsy. The child, teenager or adult, has switched-off, and gone into automatic pilot, usually because of pressure or anxiety. The child wakes normally, with no recall of the night's events.

In adults, the problem may have occurred in childhood. The personality tends to be highly strung because of stress anxiety and tension. Sleep talking is usually only a passing symptom, common in adults and reflects a failure to relax profoundly at night, with troubled dreams, restless agitated sleep, because of underlying tension. Sleepwalking of children or teenagers responds well to homoeopathy and should be treated lightly, with a minimum of attention or comment. At the same time, try to ascertain the major focus of any anxiety.

Character traits which aggravate the condition
The underlying personality is too intense, with high levels of anxiety, shyness, and a tendency to withdraw.

Practical steps to improve things
Discuss feelings more openly, especially fears about change. If you feel at all vulnerable, talk about it.

Remedies to consider:-

Aconitum   Fear, restless agitation, and emotional shock are some of the features which undermine a relaxed sleep pattern. The face is usually red. Fears about death or the future are other indications for the remedy.

Ignatia   The symptoms are part of a dissociated depressed state, often a reaction to a recent loss, acute grief, or a mourning reaction.

Kali brom   He sleeps very deeply, almost in a hypnotic state. The nights are terrifying, with teeth grinding.

Natrum mur   There is a combination of tearful depression and anxiety with a dissociated state of mind. All symptoms are worse for sympathy, consolation, or contact with others.

Pulsatilla   The state of mind is variable and contrasting throughout the day. Extremely dramatic features are characteristic, and he feels unable to relax at night. Sleeps with the hands held above the head.

Stramonium   Snores, then wakes up screaming and terrified.

SMOKING

Smoking is a damaging addictive habit which is harmful to the smoker, undermining health and vitality, and damaging to those in his environment, especially young children. The habit reflects pressure, tension and stress, although this is often denied. The typical compulsive smoker usually asserts that he only smokes from enjoyment and the pleasure it gives. He tends to deny that he smokes because he is tense and wound-up, or cannot relax and cope otherwise. In teenagers, particularly young females, it is used as a symbol of freedom from adult controls, independence, and sexual maturity. Pipe smoking is a different approach to underlying stress tension, related to satisfactions from biting and sucking. Smoking is one of the major sources of illness in every society. It can encourage the harmful repression of emotions, rather than a free and open discussion, at the same time denying an outlet for aggressive feelings, although these remain within the system. It is a high-risk habit at any age, and now considered to be a major factor in heart disease, cancer of the lung, stomach, bladder, and throat.

Character traits which aggravate the condition
The underlying personality is tense, restless and irritable, usually doing too much and under pressure and strain, most of which is self-generated.

Practical steps to improve things
Clarify the times of day when you start to become tense, and try to lessen it. Also clarify your underlying feelings, perhaps fear or anxiety about change. Look at the times when you do not smoke and try to extend these. Relax or meditate regularly.

Remedies to consider:-

Bryonia This remedy is particularly useful for a dry smokers cough, usually worse in the morning.

Nux vomica There is a combination of depression and short-fuse irritability. Both smoking and alcohol are taken to excess, causing the chronic indigestion and constipation problems.

Tabacum A useful remedy to help when trying to stop smoking. It also relieves many of the side-effects of the tobacco habit.

Tuberculinum Indicated for restless, overactive energy, always wanting to be on the move and travelling. Body weight is low, the skin pale and anaemic looking. Recurrent chest weakness is characteristic, with a dry persistent morning cough.

SUSPICION AND MISTRUST

Trust is vital to the success of any relationship, and basic to confidence. It is essential for relaxation and ease, also for healthy psychological growth. The basis of trust normally occurs in the young baby as part of the early infant-mother bonding experience, when the child develops the foundations of closeness, trust and self-reliability, a sense of continuity and contentment, which is usually only broken when weaning occurs.

Although weaning is unwelcome to the child, it does not normally dispel the basic layers of trust or the good experience, which have been built up. Without basic trust, there is lack of ease and relaxation. You may feel more hesitant or uncertain, tending to be on the defensive, wary or fearful, keeping others at a safe distance. Where loss of trust occurs as a result of an acute accident, physical assault, or divorce, all the psychological barriers may be reinforced. Suspicion and mistrust may be associated with an acute loss, separation, or rejection, frequently occurring in early childhood. For some, the early bonding experience was not satisfactory or the birth traumatic. The infant may have been premature, kept in an intensive care unit, the mother depressed, or even psychotic, in some cases, the child rejected, abused, unwanted, or abandoned.

Character traits which aggravate the condition
Envy, suspicion, hostility, may have been present
since childhood and associated with hurt, rejection, or abuse.

Practical steps to improve things
Talk more openly about your feelings and try to build a bridge of trust between yourself and others.

Remedies to consider:-

Arsenicum

A loner, who does not trust anyone, not even himself. Precise, controlled and obsessional, others are kept at a distance. Restless anguish, fear and depression are marked. Often worse in the early night hours.

Causticum

He is sensitive, with a nervous irritability, often persistently silent for long periods.

Cicuta virosa

Indifferent to others, he lacks confidence and is very mistrustful and suspicious.

Lachesis

The mood is variable. At times he may be quite lively, talkative and communicative, then developing doubts, becoming suspicious, mistrustful, jealous or fearful. Insecurity is the basic problem.

Natrum mur

The mood is one of anxious depression, tearfulness, and despair. Prefers to be alone, and always aggravated by consolation. Mood irritability is marked. Salt is craved. Aggravated by sea air. Exhaustion is marked.

SWEATING

Sweating tends to occur when the emotional system becomes overheated with uncontrollable emotions, usually panic, rage, or fear. A man mislaid a small parcel he had been asked to post. He started to panic and became drenched in sweat, fearing a reprimand, disapproval or public ridicule. The problem tends to occur when an emotional situation is out of control, one which cannot be immediately resolved, even in fantasy. Thoughts of what might happen or could have happened cause a surge of adrenalin and fear because of the panic reaction. If the fear is sustained, it can lead to burn-up of the whole nervous system, causing hot or cold sweats. The underlying psychological mechanism is often an acute flight back into infantile passivity (regression), which adds to feelings of vulnerability.

Sweating can be severe when the life-style is too neat, orderly and controlled. The inability to immediately resolve an emotional situation, can lead to further agitation and fear.

Character traits which aggravate the condition
Anxiety is due to lack of confidence, fearing others and particularly new situations. Social skills are often weak or non-existent because of an over-protected upbringing.

Practical steps to improve things
Aim to be more relaxed with others, concentrating less on how you look or feel, whether you will be liked or a success, and more concerned with being natural and yourself, making new friends and contacts. Vary your social experiences more, and mix with people and groups of all ages. Talk more openly about the problem.

Remedies to consider:-

Calcarea

For chilly exhaustion, flabby and overweight, sweats profusely on the head and hands, yet craving heat. Fear and anxiety are marked, with withdrawal from others into obsessional repetitive behaviour. There is a sour-tasting chronic indigestion problem. All symptoms are better for heat.

China

There is a profuse, oily, cold sweat over the whole body which alternates with burning heat.

Ipecacuanha

The sweating is associated with nausea and often vomiting. The mood is one of irritability. He is usually overweight, constantly complaining of feeling tired or exhausted. All symptoms are aggravated by moist warm air.

Mercurius

A remedy for states of collapse with trembling and profuse sweating. Symptoms are worse at night, from the heat of the bed, and from cold, damp conditions.

Silicea

There is offensive sweating of the feet, associated with lack of vital energy, always feeling cold. He lacks drive, confidence and initiative. Infections tend to recur.

TENSION STATES

Stress tension can cause considerable physical as well as psychological pain and discomfort. It often mimics other illnesses, in this way heightening anxiety, especially if there is fear of cancer or heart disease. Symptoms may occur in any part of the body, but are particularly frequent in the neck (stiffness, pain, twitching); scalp (pain, sensitivity, or tenderness), shoulder (a frozen shoulder); chest (often sharp localised areas of pain, as if a nail is being driven in); back (mainly low back pain or aching discomfort); limbs (stiffness or pain), hands or feet (tremor, swelling or pain). Tension can also cause purely psychological distress, with an unbearable sense of anguish in the solar plexus (upper abdominal region), fullness and a sense of oppression in the heart region, a rapid pulse, headache, palpitations. Other symptoms include:- indigestion, constipation or diarrhoea, pain or spasm of the lower abdomen (irritable bowel syndrome), sexual problems, period problems (mainly pain or irregularity), and often severe mood irritability.

Character traits which aggravate the condition
Emotions are kept locked up tightly inside as if they would erupt or burst out uncontrollably, adding to anxiety. A tendency to be shy and lacking confidence.

Practical steps to improve things
Spend part of each day relaxing deeply. Try to be quiet avoiding the accumulation of tension within the body. Express your moods and feelings, and be more natural and spontaneous. If there is a physical problem, try to see when the symptoms started, and the stress situation which first triggered their appearance.

Remedies to consider:-

Arsenicum
For a tense, agitated, restless, state of mind. He is thin, tired, fussy, neat and obsessional. All symptoms are worse after midnight, from damp cold air.

Gelsemium
A remedy for mild tension states, with apathy. It is often indicated for a more dramatic type of temperament, with phobic anxiety problems, especially talking in public.

Lycopodium
There is a facade of pseudo-maturity covering-up tension and low self-esteem. Accident-prone, and always in a hurry, creates a chain of disasters whenever he tries to be helpful. He is often tense with his peers and more at home with young children or the elderly. Concentration is poor because he is easily distracted.

Natrum mur
A remedy for severe stress problems, with depression, anguish, and marked exhaustion. Feels worse for sympathy, or contact with others.

Nux vomica
Irritability is marked, with impatience and depression.

TRANQUILLISER DEPENDENCY

This is a common side-effect of tranquilliser medication, especially the benzodiazepines, causing disturbing symptoms whenever any attempt is made to stop or cut down on dosage. Anguish, tension, apathy, palpitations, a slow pulse, dry skin, nausea, malaise, may occur, reinforcing any underlying lack of confidence. The symptoms may cause panic, and oblige the patient to increase the dosage, often to continue taking the tranquilliser for years, or indefinitely. The reactions may be more severe than the psychological condition requiring treatment in the first place, often more distressing or prolonged. Reactions tend to occur because anxiety levels increase as the tranquilliser dosage is reduced. Typically reactions include depression, panic attacks, insomnia, anxiety, sweating, a feeling of impending collapse. After stopping the drug, symptoms may persist for months or years.

Homoeopathy combined with focal counselling can usually fully resolve the problem.

Character traits which aggravate the condition
There is a tendency to be over-dependent in every aspect of life, especially on a medication, but also an unfulfilling job or unsatisfactory relationship.

Practical steps to improve things
Try to slowly reduce your dosage, carefully looking at the emotions which are released without letting panic take over. Talk in greater depth about your feelings. Look at the situation which started your need for tranquillisers and try to clarify how you have changed since then, and are feeling stronger.

Remedies to consider:-

Argentum nit　　Fear and apprehension are marked, with many phobic problems which are not always quickly resolved. Lack of self-confidence leads to a renewal of tranquilliser dependency problems. Anxiety and fear may re-appear as soon as the dosage is cut down.

Natrum mur　　Because of the extreme weakness, depression, anxiety, and tearful moods, he is prone to become addicted to tranquillisers. The amount of help derived from them is variable, and often minimal in the long term. But stopping seems an impossibility because of tension, anguish and fear, as soon as they are reduced.

Silicea　　This remedy is useful when the underlying problem is lack of drive and determination. There is a profound lack of self-confidence. He is constantly searching for props and short-cuts. The ultimate cure is a profound re-thinking of attitudes, becoming more open and spontaneous.

The specific tranquilliser in potency

VERTIGO

Stress vertigo is an unpleasant sensation of dizziness. Objects in the environment appear to rotate, feel unreliable, or seem to move erratically. Sometimes they seem to be giving way, causing a swaying movement. This is often felt on one particular side of the head or body, undermining confidence and movement, limiting travel. There is a feeling of insecurity because of the lack of co-ordination. It may be accompanied by nausea, and particularly causes problems when walking or travelling, for example by car. Vertigo can also occur after getting up too quickly, suddenly turning the head, or when caught off-balance.

Vertigo is sometimes associated with noises in the head (tinnitus), headache, weakness, nausea, and malaise.

The major cause of stress vertigo is nearly always a build-up of emotional tension and pressure, often accumulated over a period of months or years. Physical causes of vertigo include high blood-pressure, problems of the spine in the neck region, or an acute infection.

Character traits which aggravate the condition
There is a tendency to worry unduly about minor matters, especially anticipating future problems.
Often too much emphasis is put on neatness and order, with fussy obsessional tendencies.

Practical steps to improve things
Aim to be more at ease with yourself and others. Deal with problems as they arise, not before. Reduce tension by not imposing high standards which are impossible to ever achieve and which cause anxiety.

Remedies to consider:-

Aconitum   For states of restless agitation. Vertigo is usually worse on getting up, or sudden head movements.

Cocculus   For symptoms associated with nausea, and headache at the back of the head and upper neck region. It is worse for movement.

Gelsemium   The head feels heavy, the vertigo seems to spread around the whole head area, but improved by fresh air and walking. Apathy with no desire for social contacts and fearful of appearing in public.

Opium   The head feels light-headed and dull. The vertigo is worse on first waking, from heat, any sudden shock or fear.

Pulsatilla   For variable symptoms, but always worse for heat. There are tearful mood swings, and thirst is usually absent.

Salicylic acid Vertigo is often associated with rheumatic pains. There is a tendency to fall to the left side. Headache and tinnitus may also occur (Meniere's Syndrome).

INDEX

189

OTHER INSIGHT PUBLICATIONS

HOMOEOPATHY

Understanding Homoeopathy (£6.95)

The revised second edition of this comprehensive book explains in clear, simple terms the basic principles of homoeopathy, which can be readily understood by the beginner. The author outlines the approach, indications, and choice of remedies for the common health problems of the family.

Talking About Homoeopathy (£4.95)

An invaluable reference book for anyone wishing to understand homoeopathy. The book covers a variety of topics of general interest which offer a deeper understanding and a more challenging awareness of homoeopathy, its indications, potential, and scope of action.

The Principles, Art and Practice of Homoeopathy (£6.95)

A book which explains in simple language the principles of homoeopathic practice and prescribing. It includes chapters on :- Dosage, Potency, First and Second Prescriptions, Homoeopathic History Taking, and The Consultation. A second section is concerned with Constitutional Prescribing and the role of homoeopathy in the treatment of Cancer.

PSYCHOLOGY

Emotional Health (£5.95)

A unique and major study of the most common emotional problems facing society in the twentieth century. It identifies their causes and symptoms, and then explains the most practical, self-help steps that can be taken to solve them. Simple guidelines are given in order to promote healthier attitudes, changes in specific problem areas, and better psychological perspectives.

Personal Growth and Creativity (£4.95)

A guide to the most effective ways to stimulate and develop personal creativity in order to bring about positive change in outlook. The book offers practical guidelines that will lead to constructive results.

RISKS OF MODERN LIVING

The Side-Effects Book (£16.95)

This books describes in detail the most common hazards of our pressurised society, the props used, and their risk to health. Chapters include: Developmental Stages of life, Stress and the Home, Sexuality, Over-The-Counter Drugs, Health Products and Vitamins, Medically Prescribed Drugs, Surgical and Cosmetic Procedures, Immunisation, Food and Diet, Social Addictions, Holidays and the Sun, Travel, Sport, Occupations, Animals and Plants, Household Products, Pesticides, Drugs of Dependence and Misuse, Pollution.

Please send a s.a.e. for list of other available titles.

192